**Emna Bokri**
**Traki Mazouni**
**Nesrine Hasni**

# Interventional Neuroradiology: Economic evaluation

**Emna Bokri**
**Traki Mazouni**
**Nesrine Hasni**

# Interventional Neuroradiology: Economic evaluation

## Interventional neuroradiology

**ScienciaScripts**

**Imprint**

Any brand names and product names mentioned in this book are subject to trademark, brand or patent protection and are trademarks or registered trademarks of their respective holders. The use of brand names, product names, common names, trade names, product descriptions etc. even without a particular marking in this work is in no way to be construed to mean that such names may be regarded as unrestricted in respect of trademark and brand protection legislation and could thus be used by anyone.

Cover image: www.ingimage.com

This book is a translation from the original published under ISBN 978-620-6-71920-5.

Publisher:
Sciencia Scripts
is a trademark of
Dodo Books Indian Ocean Ltd. and OmniScriptum S.R.L publishing group

120 High Road, East Finchley, London, N2 9ED, United Kingdom
Str. Armeneasca 28/1, office 1, Chisinau MD-2012, Republic of Moldova, Europe
Printed at: see last page
**ISBN: 978-620-8-05522-6**

# *Contents*

# INTRODUCTION

Imaging-guided interventions or interventional radiology aim to improve the efficiency and precision of medical procedures, whatever the pathology to be treated, as well as patient safety and comfort. The field of interventional radiology today covers all medical and surgical specialties, including neurosurgery, with a constant increase in the number of procedures[1].

Advances in medical imaging, technique and device technology have broadened the spectrum of cerebro-medullary vascular pathologies treatable by the neuroendovascular route[2]. Since the publication in the 2000s of several studies focusing on interventional neuroradiology and its contribution to the treatment of neurovascular pathologies, the management of vascular malformations and intracranial aneurysms has changed[3-6].

Interventional neuroradiology today represents a major field of innovation, responding to strong societal demand for increasingly effective, yet less invasive treatments[1].

This neuroradiological approach is more marked in France than in other countries. Literature and studies on the pharmacoeconomics and cost-effectiveness of endovascular treatment in interventional neuroradiology have grown exponentially in recent years.

In Tunisia, this endovascular treatment technique is undergoing gradual but slow development, hampered by economic factors among other factors.

In this context, we have carried out a study at the Institut National de Neurologie (INN), the main aim of which is to evaluate the overall cost of an interventional neuroradiology procedure.

# 1. BIBLIOGRAPHIC REVIEW

*"Interventional Radiology (IR) includes all invasive medical procedures aimed at the diagnosis and/or treatment of a pathology and performed under the guidance and control of an imaging device (X-ray, ultrasound, scanner, magnetic resonance imaging)"*[7].

Interventional vascular neuroradiology uses cerebral angiography to diagnose and treat vascular pathologies of the central nervous system[8]. Angiography is a radiological examination of blood vessels. In some cases, it is possible to convert diagnostic angiography into endovascular treatment by adapting the equipment to the procedure. In this case, the term "angiography" is replaced by "embolization"[8].

Embolization is a supra-selective endovascular catheterization procedure to treat a vascular malformation of the central nervous system[9].

Endovascular treatments have rapidly evolved to offer a therapeutic alternative to other approaches in many fields, including[...7,8]:

- Embolization of ruptured and unruptured cerebral aneurysms.
- Embolization of cerebral arteriovenous malformations (cerebral AVMs).
- Embolization of medullary dural arteriovenous fistulas (dAVF).
- Revascularization of occluded arteries in the event of acute stroke (cerebral thrombectomy).
- Pre-surgical embolization of certain tumors.

## 1.1 Endovascular catheterization

Embolization procedures are generally performed in an interventional neuroradiology suite, under general anesthetic, using a microcatheter[10]. The first step in catheterization is endovascular access, usually via the femoral route. This allows easy access to all cerebral vessels. When vaginal catheterization is not possible, direct puncture of the carotid artery remains an alternative[10].

In the second stage, a stent is inserted into the common femoral artery. A carrier catheter is then inserted, and taken up to the cervical vessels: carotid or vertebral arteries [10].

A microcatheter is then inserted into the supporting catheter. The tip of this microcatheter, fitted with a radiopaque index, is guided with the aid of a microguide and under fluoroscopic guidance (X-rays) to the target artery[10].

Depending on the arteriovenous pathology being treated, several devices or materials can be deployed or injected through the microcatheter[11].

The **figure 1** the various stages of endovascular catheterization using femoral puncture.

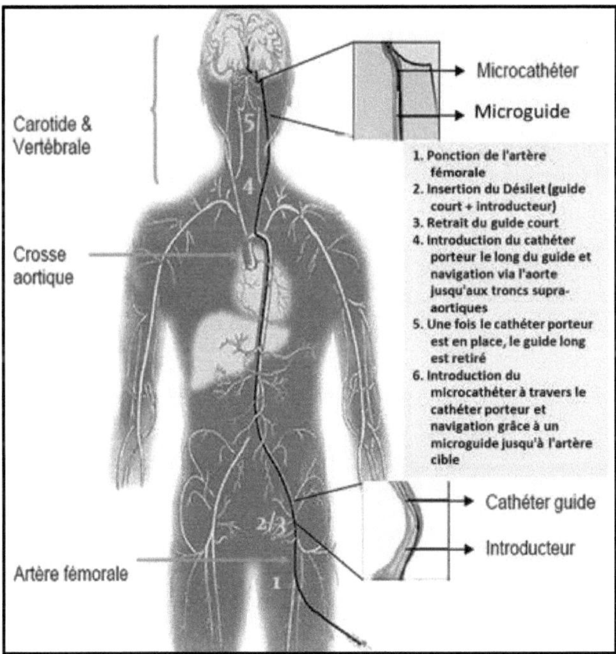


**Figure 1Endovascular catheterization procedure via the femoral artery [12]**

## 1.2. Intracranial aneurysm

### 1.2.1. Definition

Intracranial aneurysms are localized dilatations of the intracranial arteries, progressively forming in areas of reduced resistance in the arterial wall. Aneurysms consist of a pocket that implants itself on the artery at the level of the neck (**Fig. 2**). These pockets vary in size, with [13]:

- Small aneurysms less than 5 mm in diameter.
- Medium to large aneurysms with diameters of between 6 and 25 mm.
- Giant aneurysms with a diameter greater than 25 mm.

And they are classified according to their shape:

- Or localized, bag-shaped pockets formed by regular, rounded dilatation.
- Or long dilations that increase vessel diameter.

These forms are known as saccular aneurysms and fusiform aneurysms respectively (**Figure 2**) [13].

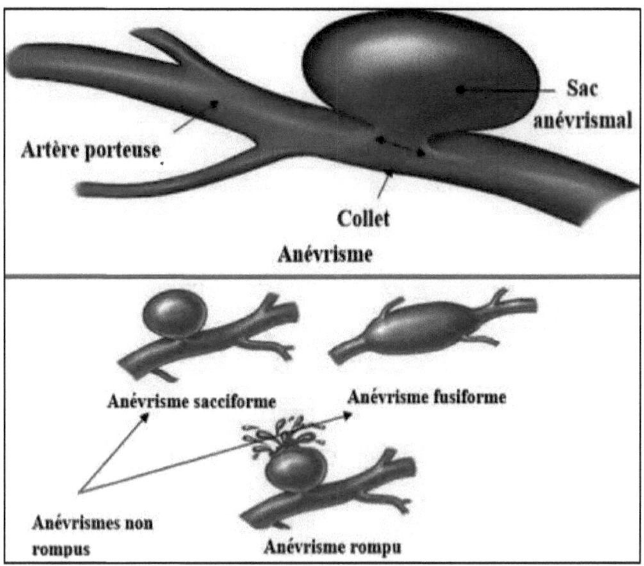


**Figure 2Intracranial aneurysm and its various forms [14]**

Intracranial aneurysms tend to increase in volume under the influence of hemodynamic factors. This volume expansion leads to a weakening of the aneurysm's wall and to rupture. This is why aneurysm rupture is the most frequent means of discovery, and also the most dramatic. For this reason, aneurysms are classified according to their status, i.e. ruptured, latent unruptured and symptomatic unruptured[15].

Most aneurysms are saccular, and are most often located at the branching points of the arteries of the circle of Willis. Common sites for saccular aneurysms include the anterior communicating artery, the posterior communicating artery, the internal carotid artery, the middle cerebral artery and the bifurcation of the basilar artery [16].

Saccular aneurysms are more likely to rupture than fusiform aneurysms [17].

Although the exact pathogenesis of intracranial aneurysm remains unknown, several hypotheses have highlighted the contribution of maladaptive vascular remodeling triggered by hemodynamic stress and inflammatory response, a chain of events that would ultimately damage blood vessel walls and lead to intracranial aneurysm [13].

Intracranial aneurysms are considered sporadically acquired lesions, although a rare familial form has been described. It is estimated that 5-40% of patients with autosomal dominant polycystic kidney disease have intracranial aneurysms, and 10-30% of patients have multiple aneurysms[16,18].

Aneurysms are classified and qualified according to the diameter of the aneurysm sac, the neck and the state of rupture (**Table I**).

**Table ICriteria for classifying aneurysms [13,15]**

| Aneurysm condition | Broken | |
|---|---|---|
| | Unbroken | |
| **Aneurysm size** | | |
| Aneurysmal sac diameter | Diameter ≤ 5 mm | Small |
| | 5 mm < diameter ≤ 25 mm | Medium to large |
| | Diameter > 25 mm | Giant |
| **Collet** | | |
| Neck diameter | Diameter < half of the largest bag diameter | Small |
| | Diameter ≥ half of the largest bag diameter | Large |

The aim of treating ruptured and unruptured aneurysms is the same: occlude the aneurysm to prevent and/or stop bleeding. Aneurysm occlusion can be achieved in two ways: surgically, using clips, or endovascularly, by filling the aneurysm sac with coils (**Fig. 3**). Endovascular coiling is a less invasive procedure than surgical clipping [19].

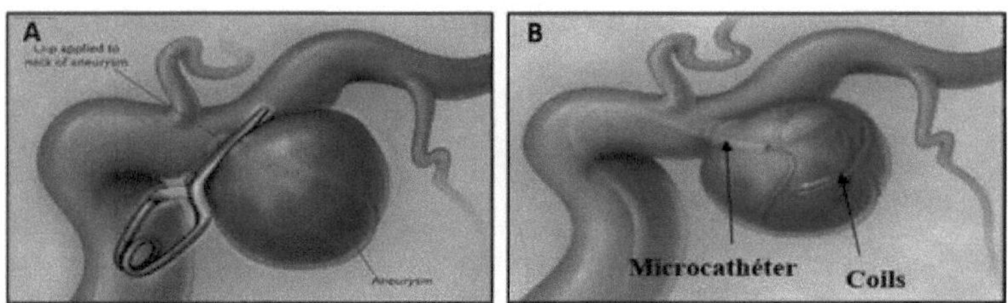


**Figure 3Surgical clipping (A) and coilingendovascular clipping (B) [20]**

## 1.2.2. Coils

The spiral-shaped coils are made from a platinum alloy that is perfectly compatible with MRI. They come in a wide variety of sizes, shapes and flexibilities to suit all types of aneurysm. The smallest coils measure 1 mm in diameter, while the largest are over 20 mm [21].

The coils not only allow mechanical occlusion of the aneurysm by endovascular filling of the aneurysm sac, but also induce thrombosis, local fibrosis and subsequent parietal scarring Once unwound in the vessel, the coil remains attached to the guide, enabling the operator to reintegrate it into the microcatheter if necessary. It is therefore possible to change the position of the coil, or remove it completely to insert another of a different diameter or length[22].

Coils are characterized by[23]:

- **Their size**: the length and diameter of the coil and the diameter of the ellipse. The appropriate coil size is chosen during embolization, after assessing the size of the aneurysm.
- **Their shape (figure 4)**: 2D and 3D: 2D helical shape, from 1$^{\text{ère}}$ generation, used for aneurysm filling. And the 3D spherical shape, from 2$^{\text{ème}}$ generation, used to form a cage in the aneurysm and improve subsequent filling with 2D coils.
- **Their flexibility**: rigid (to form the cage), intermediate and flexible (to fill the aneurysm).
- **Their detachment system:** Electrolytic, mechanical and electro-thermal.
- **The presence or absence of an active substance**.

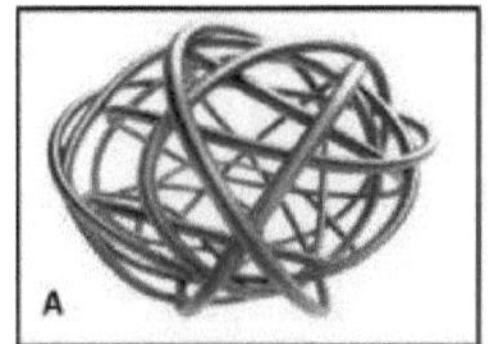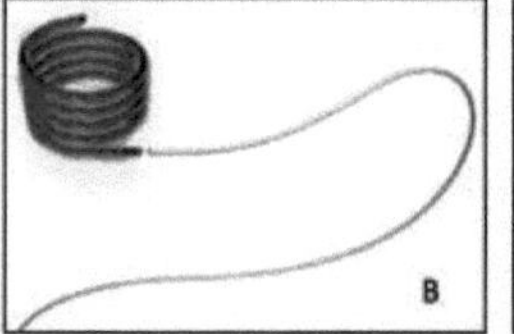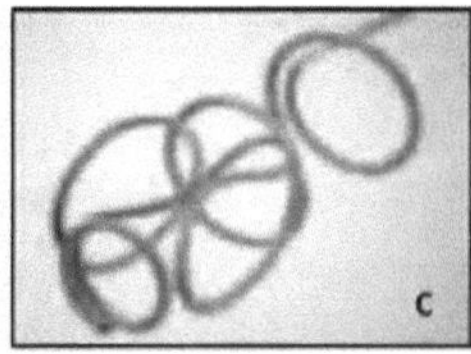

**Figure 43D coil (A), 2D coil (B) and 2D/3D/2D coil (C) [9]**

### 1.2.3. Endovascular treatment of intracranial aneurysms

Embolization of intracranial aneurysms is certainly the procedure that has had the greatest impact on interventional neuroradiology. The principle is to reach inside the aneurysm sac using a microcatheter to drop coils of various sizes and shapes to reduce the amount of blood and prevent it from filling the aneurysm[22].

Once the tip of the microcatheter has been placed in the aneurysm sac, and after verification at different incidences, the first coil can be inserted, the diameter and length of which will be chosen according to the angioarchitecture of the sac [24].

Once the coil is in place, and after angiographic control, it is released electrically or mechanically. If necessary, additional coils are inserted and released to fill the aneurysm sac as completely as possible[24].

The challenge is to occlude the entire sac without leaving any permeability at the neck and without occluding the supporting artery. A metal ball is formed and condensed until the contrast medium no longer opacifies the aneurysm on follow-up angiography (**Fig. 5**). The procedure is stopped when the aneurysm is completely occluded[24].

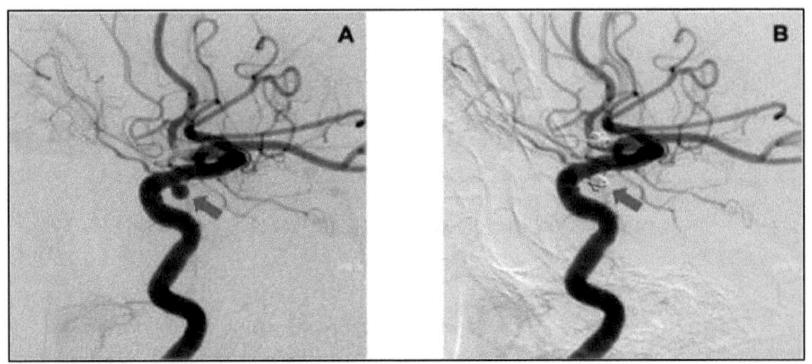

**Figure 5Angiography before aneurysm embolization (A)
and angiography after aneurysm
embolization (B)
[Photo taken at INN
Neuroradiology Department].**

There are currently four techniques for aneurysm embolization[25]:

- **The *coiling* technique:** this involves simple embolization using coils, small metal springs which fill part of the aneurysm sac to reduce blood flow and induce thrombosis. It is intended for narrow-neck aneurysms [25].

- **The balloon *remodeling* technique (figure 6):** used to treat wide-neck aneurysms. The coils are deployed in the aneurysm sac, with the lumen of the supporting vessel protected by a balloon [26].

  The non-detachable balloon is first placed temporarily in the carrier vessel in front of the aneurysm neck. We then perform a super-selective microcatheterization of the aneurysm. The non-detachable balloon is inflated in front of the aneurysm neck, temporarily occluding the neck and the supporting vessel. Under the protection of the balloon, coils are then deposited in the aneurysm sac [27]. After placement of each coil, but before detachment, the balloon is deflated to test the stability of the material in the sac. If no displacement is observed, the coil is detached. If, however, there are undesirable changes in the position of the coil, it is retrieved and another attempt is made, either with the same coil, or with one of a different diameter[27].

- **The *coiling stenting* technique (figure 6):** the number of indications for stent placement in the carrier vessel is increasing, enabling embolization of aneurysms without collar or at high risk of recanalization that were previously inaccessible to endovascular treatment. Coil embolization is performed through the mesh of the stent previously deployed in the carrier vessel **[25]**.

- **The *flow-diverter stenting* technique (Figure 7):**the use of this device for the treatment of ruptured aneurysms carries a higher risk of thromboembolic and hemorrhagic complications**[28]**.

  This technique is therefore reserved for aneurysms with a very wide neck, or without a neck, which cannot be treated by coils alone or by surgery. *Flow-diverters* are recently developed self-expanding stents featuring a very tight braid that redirects flow to occlude the aneurysm without the need for additional coils**[29]**.

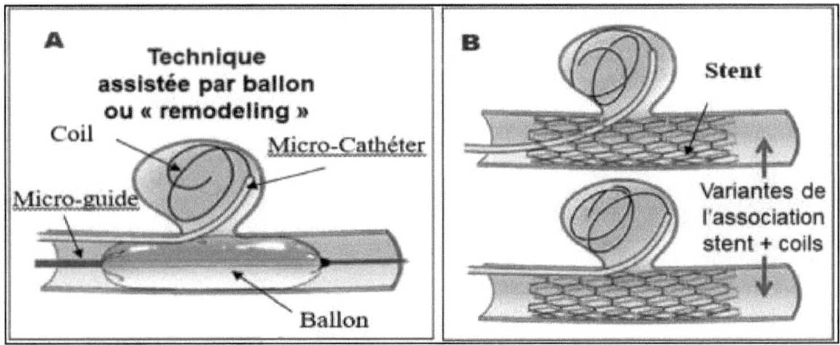


**Figure 6*Remodeling* technique (A) and *stenting* technique (B) [30]**

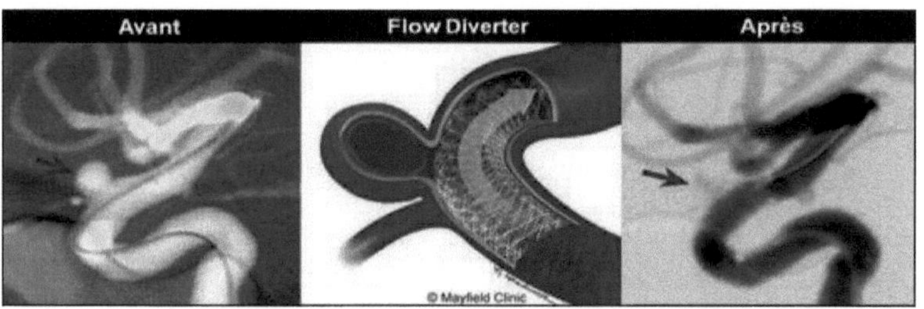

**Figure 7***Flow-diverter stenting* **technique[30]**

## 1.3 Arteriovenous malformations

### 1.3.1. Definition

Arteriovenous malformations (AVMs) of the brain are congenital or acquired anomalies of the blood vessels due to poor development of the capillary network. They are characterized by abnormal communications between the arterial and venous sectors, through the vascular bundle known as the nidus (**figure 8**) [31].

The most common symptoms of an AVM are cerebral hemorrhage, seizures, transient neurological deficit and headaches, including migraines [32].

In cases where the risk of bleeding is considered high enough to warrant intervention, treatment options include surgical resection, radiosurgery or embolization (or a combination of all three, in some cases)[31].

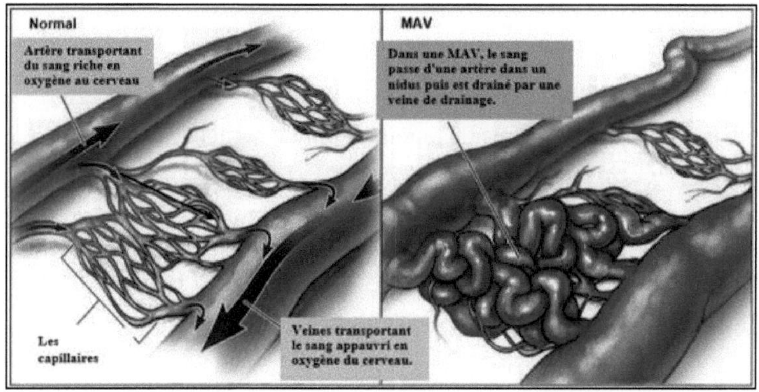


**Figure 8Normal cerebral blood flow VS blood flow
in a cerebral AVM [after 33]**

## 1.3.2. Embolic agents

For the embolization of AVMs and dural arteriovenous fistulas, two embolic agents classified as medical devices can be used:

**- Onyx 18®** : Onyx® is a medical device composed of biocompatible polymers containing ethylene vinyl alcohol (EVOH) dissolved in an organic solvent, dimethyl sulfoxide (DMSO), and suspended micronized tantalum powder used as contrast for fluoroscopic visualization [34].

It is a liquid embolic agent used for the embolization of cerebral arteriovenous malformations. The solidification process is slow and proceeds from the outside in. This technique enables slower, more controllable injection and should result in more effective filling of the AVM nidus[35].

**- Glubran® 2: Glubran** surgical glue® 2or N-Butyl-2-cyanoacrylate (nBCA) is a clear, fluid liquid used for embolization since the 1980s [...9]. This glue is mixed with tantalum powder or ethiodized oil to obtain a two-component embolic agent. The added agent prolongs polymerization time, opacifies the liquid agent and enables it to be visualized under fluoroscopy[36].

### 1.3.3. Endovascular treatment of arteriovenous malformations

Embolization is one of three therapeutic approaches that can be used either to treat AVMs definitively, or as a complementary or preceding step to the other methods. Particularly in the case of large arteriovenous malformations, embolization is used preoperatively to progressively reduce blood flow and the size of the malformation prior to definitive surgical resection **(Fig.9)[6]**.

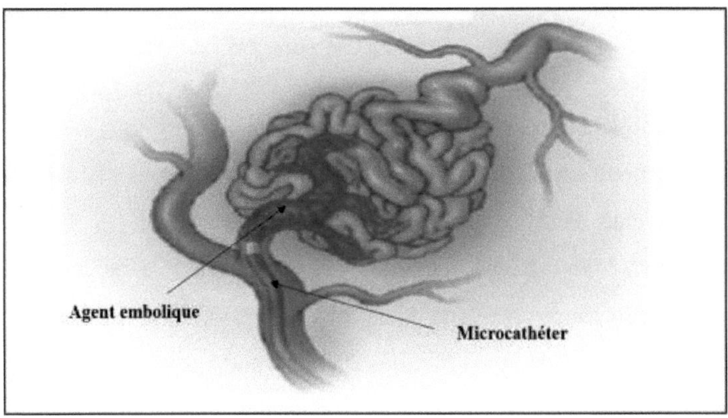


**Figure 9Endovascular treatment of arteriovenous malformations [after 6]**

Endovascular treatment of arteriovenous malformations is achieved by injecting liquid embolic agents such as Onyx® through a compatible microcatheter. The procedure requires super-selective catheterization of the arteries feeding the AVM, with the aim of filling the nidus and occluding the feeding vessels, while preserving the collateral vessels of the adjacent normal brain **(Fig.10)[6]**.

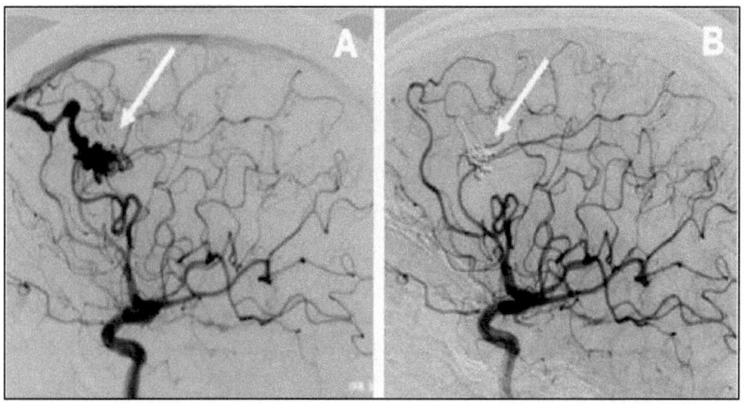

**Figure 10Angiography of an AVM before (A) and after (B) embolization [Photo taken at the INN Neuroradiology Department].**

## 1.4. Spinal dural arteriovenous fistulas

### 1.4.1. Definition

Spinal dural arteriovenous fistulas (SDAFs) represent a subset of a heterogeneous group of spinal vascular malformations that can cause acute, subacute or chronic spinal cord dysfunction. Unlike AVMs, there is a direct communication (shunt) between a radiculo-medullary artery and a drainage vein without interposition of a malformative nidus[37].

Two treatment modalities are possible: endovascular or surgical[38].

### 1.4.2. Endovascular treatment of dural arteriovenous fistulas

Endovascular treatment of FAVd is achieved by injection, through a compatible microcatheter, of liquid embolic agents such as n-butylcyanoacrylate (nBCA) or Onyx®. The procedure requires super-selective catheterization of the arteries supplying the fistula, with the aim of filling and occluding the fistulous connection [39].

## 1.5. Cerebrovascular accident

### 1.5.1. Definition

Ischemic stroke results from the obstruction of cerebral arteries by a clot, which leads to a loss of oxygenation in downstream brain tissue, ultimately resulting in neuronal cell death and irreversible neurological deficit[...40].

If blockage is eliminated before significant tissue damage ensues, reperfusion of hypoperfused tissue can reverse or compensate for this risk of injury[41].

The timing of the procedure is a critical factor: in general, the longer it takes to block a cerebral artery, the more irreversible cell death occurs[41].

### 1.5.2. Mechanical thrombectomy of ischemic stroke

Mechanical thrombectomy is a technique used to remove a blood clot obstructing a cerebral artery, the cause of an ischemic stroke, in order to restore blood flow[42].

The thrombectomy procedure involves puncturing the femoral artery, catheterizing up to the obstructed brain artery and retrieving and extracting the clot with a revascularization device, which is then removed[43].

Mechanical revascularization devices can be divided into two groups according to their mechanisms of action on the thrombus[44]:

- Clot removal systems, which require deployment by crossing the site of arterial occlusion (distal catheterization mechanism)(**Figure11**).

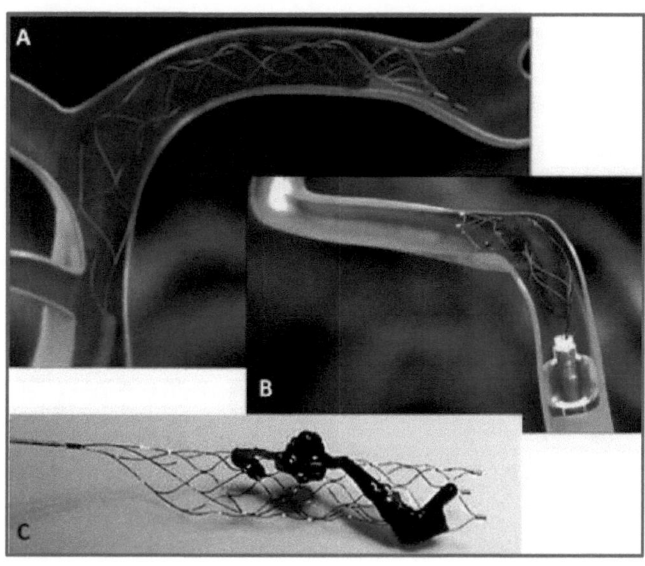

**Figure 11Mechanical thrombectomy using a retractable stent [45]**
*A) Deployment of the retractable stent within the clot. B) Removal of the impacted clot from the*
*stent. C) Clot withdrawn into stent mesh.*

- Thrombus aspiration systems to revascularize the occluded vessel, positioned upstream of the occlusion site (ADAPT:*A Direct Aspiration first Pass* Technique) (**Fig.12**).

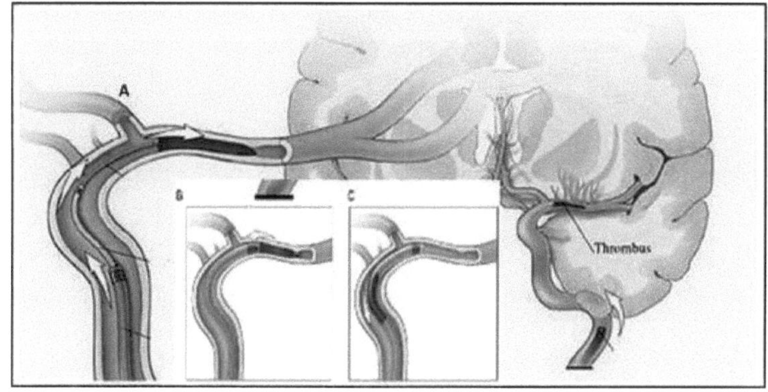

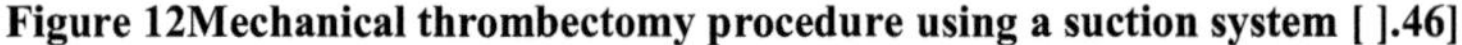

**Figure 12Mechanical thrombectomy procedure using a suction system [ ].46]**

# 2. MATERIALS AND METHODS

## 2.1. Study characteristics

This is a prospective pharmacoeconomic study that looked at patients who underwent an interventional neuroradiology (INN) procedure at the Neuroradiology Department of the National Neurological Institute from March 19, 2019 to June 19, 2019.Patients were followed up from the day of the INN procedure to the date of discharge from the INN.

The objectives of the study are:

- Main objective: To determine the total cost of an NRI intervention.

- Secondary objectives:

  - Identify the factors influencing variations in this total cost per patient.

  - To determine whether or not the expenses incurred in treating patients hospitalized for embolization procedures exceeded the allowances set by the French National Health Insurance Fund (Caisse Nationale d'Assurance Maladie).

### 2.1.1. Study location

The study was carried out in the Neuroradiology Department at NIN, which is divided into three main units:

- CT unit.
- Magnetic Resonance Imaging Unit.
- Interventional neuroradiology unit (**figures13 and 14**).

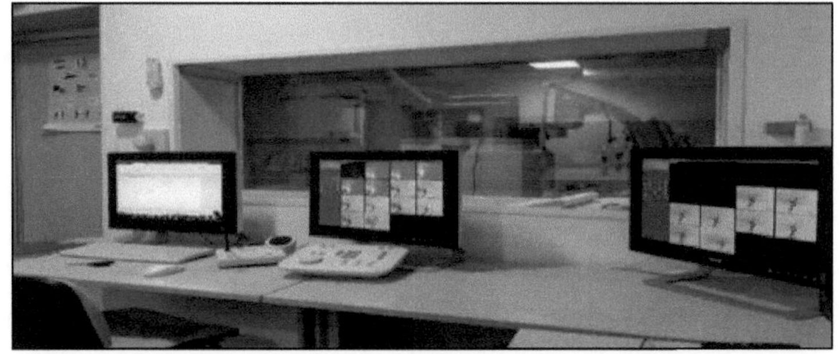

**Figure 13NRI control room at the Institute of Neurology**

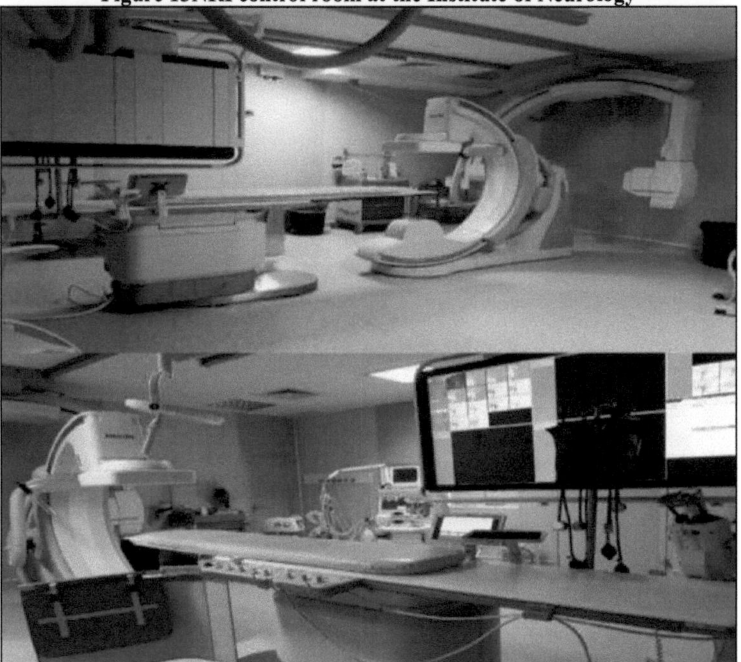

**Figure 14:Interventional neuroradiology room at INN**

The NRI unit's medical and paramedical staff consists of:

- Two radiologists specialized in interventional neuroradiology.

- A general supervisor.

- Seven senior technicians.

- Three nurses.

## 2.1.2. Study patients

INN is the only public health facility where embolization procedures for vascular malformations of the central nervous system are performed.

In the Radiology Department, the embolization procedure is either scheduled in advance or performed on an emergency basis. Following the procedure, the patient is hospitalized in one of the INN units, depending on his or her state of health.

### 2.1.2.1. Inclusion criteria

All patients who had undergone an NRI procedure and had presented:

- A small to large aneurysm, ruptured or unruptured.
- A MAV.
- A brain tumor.
- A FAVd.
- Intracerebral thrombosis (ischemic stroke).

### 2.1.2.2. Non-inclusion criteria

- Aneurysms whose location in the cerebral artery makes endovascular access impossible.
- Small aneurysms less than 2mm in diameter are considered non-embolizable.
- Aneurysms with very wide necks greater than 7mm.
- Patients with high blood pressure (PAS > 260 mmHg), resistant to antihypertensive drugs, during general anesthesia, allergy to iodinated contrast media, infectious syndrome with fever.

### 2.2. Embolization protocol at Institut National de Neurologie

The INN embolization protocol is shown in **figure15**.

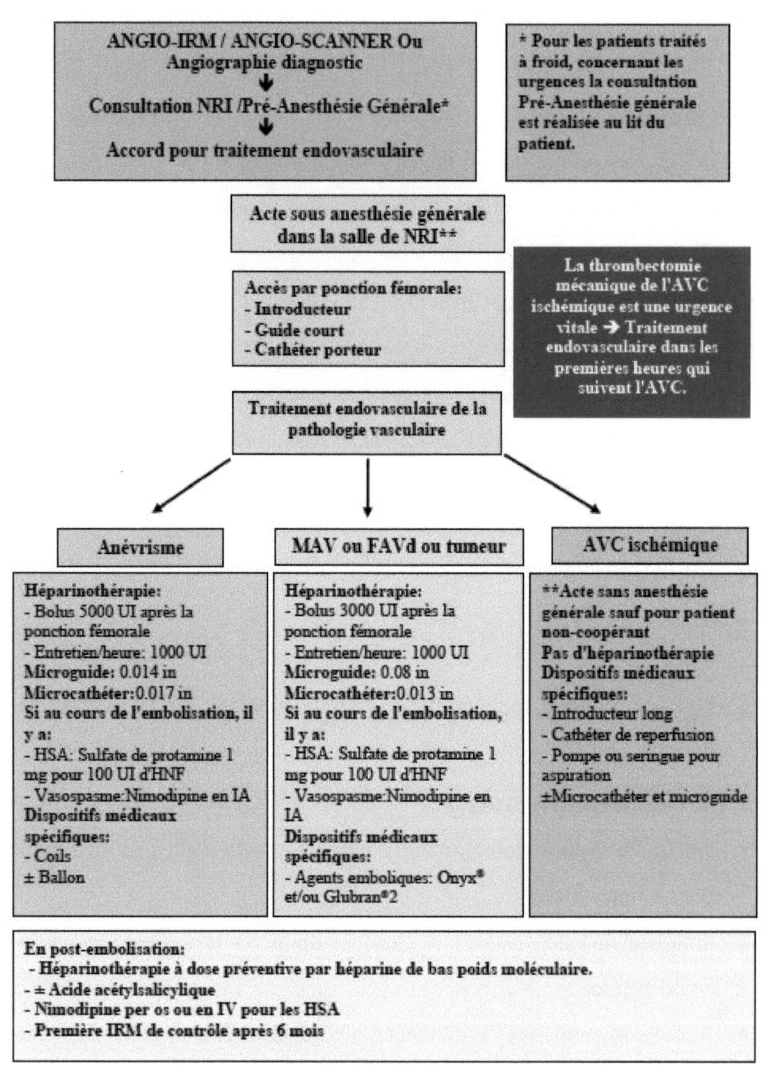


**Figure 15INN embolization protocol**

## 2.3 Study methodology

### 2.3.1. Data collection

Data were collected prospectively using a standardized data collection form (**Appendix 1**). Three types of data were collected for each patient:

- Epidemiological data: were collected from the medical record, giving each patient's surname, first name, sex, age, medical history, address, profession, type of social security coverage and diagnosis.

- Data on pharmaceutical products and medical devices used: those used during the procedure were collected by direct observation and from the neuroradiology department's traceability sheets, indicating the various drugs, non-implantable medical devices (guides, catheters, microcatheters, microguides, angiography kit, etc.) and implantable medical devices (coils and surgical glue) used.

- Pharmaceutical products and devices used during hospitalization were collected from the 24h signs on the various care units.

- Cost-accounting financial data corresponding to expenditure for the embolization room and each care unit were supplied by the finance department.

### 2.3.2. Cost analysis

### 2.3.2.1. Direct costs

Costs include all changes in resource consumption attributable to the intervention studied[47].

They are defined as the value of all resources consumed directly in its production[...47].

A distinction is made between direct medical costs and direct non-medical costs[...47].

### ❖ Direct medical costs

Direct medical costs are associated with drugs and medical or surgical care. They include the costs of drugs, medical devices, diagnostic tests, physician consultation fees and hospitalization[47].

Direct medical costs were used in the formula to calculate the total cost for each patient treated for an NRI procedure.

> **Medicines**

The same drug protocol was used for the majority of patients, except in special cases where we used antihypertensives, antiplatelet agents, corticoids and protamine sulfate.

For general anesthesia, propofol was used for induction and maintenance of sedation. Cisatracurium and fentanyl were used as muscle relaxants to facilitate intubation. Occasionally, Sevoflurane was used.

Heparin sodium was used to maintain effective anticoagulation throughout the procedure to prevent thromboembolic complications. An initial bolus of 5000 IU UFH (100 IU/kg) was administered as soon as femoral puncture was performed, followed by a maintenance dose of 20-50 IU/kg every hour to maintain effective anticoagulation[25].

The use of protamine sulfate, at a dose of 1 mg per 100 U of UFH, has sometimes been necessary to antagonize the effect of heparin, following the onset of a hemorrhagic complication[25].

Iodinated contrast media were injected intra-arterially for visualization, localization and vectoring of the area to be treated throughout the procedure.

Nimodipine, has been used as a vasodilator by intra-arterial injection in the event of severe vasospasm during embolization and post embolization at a dosage of 360 mg/d per os for 21 days in the absence of vasospasm, extended to six weeks in the event of vasospasm[48].

Drugs represent the total expenditure on drugs used, per patient, during surgery and hospitalization.

- During the procedure, the medications used by the patient were recorded by direct observation.
- During hospitalization, the medications used were collected daily from the 24h signs on the care units.

Any opened bottle is considered to have been fully consumed. With the exception of Sevoflurane and Nimodipine, their cost has been calculated per volume consumed per patient.

The valuation of medicines has been carried out using the purchase prices of products from the central pharmacy for 2018 and 2019.

> **Hospitalization costs**

These fees have been defined on the basis of the 2019 NIN annual budget granted by the Ministry of Public Health.

There are two payment plans:

- The full rate, which represents the amount to be paid by the patient per day of hospitalization. It includes medical and paramedical staff costs, medical operating expenses, hotel and general operating expenses, and depreciation.  It does not include drugs or diagnostic tests (biological analyses and medical imaging).

- The CNAM plan represents a fixed fee that patients must pay regardless of the length of their hospital stay. Unlike the full-price plan, this package includes drugs and diagnostic tests.

Hospital charges by department are shown in **tableII**.

**Table IIHospitalization costs for both plans, by hospital ward.**

| Hospitalization department | Full price | CNAM |
|---|---|---|
| Neurology | 35,000 DT/day | 65,000 DT/stay |
| Neurosurgery | 40,000 DT/day | 70,000 DT/stay |
| Resuscitation | 60,000 DT/day | 90,000 DT/stay |

For the purposes of this study, we have used the full-price plan to calculate actual hospital costs.

> **Medical and paramedical staff costs:**

These costs have been divided into 3 groups:

- Medical consultation fees set at 34 dinars. This amount was used in the formula to calculate the total cost for each patient treated for an NRI procedure.

- Medical and paramedical staff costs during the operation: These costs were accounted for using the monthly salaries of medical and paramedical staff as follows:

$$\text{Frais par heure} = \frac{(\text{salaire brut mensuel} + \text{coût employeur})}{26 \times 8}$$

*26 represents the number of working days and 8 the number of working hours per day.

For an average operating time of 4 hours, these costs were estimated at 125.320 dinars. This amount was used in the formula to calculate the total cost for each patient treated for an NRI procedure.

- Costs of medical and paramedical staff during hospitalization: these costs are already included in hospitalization costs.

> **Medical devices**

Total expenditure on medical devices (MD) includes those used, per patient, during the procedure as well as during hospitalization. Data were collected by direct observation and from the traceability sheet for the operating room and care units.

The DMs we used during the NRI procedure were divided into three groups:

**Class III DM:**

- ✓ Coils
- ✓ Embolic agents (Onyx®, Glubran®)

**Class IIb DM:**

- ✓ Désilet
- ✓ Carrier guides
- ✓ Carrier catheters
- ✓ Microguides
- ✓ Microcatheters
- ✓ Hyperform and hyperglide balls
- ✓ Peripheral catheters
- ✓ Single and armed intubation tubes, Guedel and tracheostomy cannulas
- ✓ Foley probe

**Class I DM:**

- ✓ Detailer
- ✓ Angiography kit
- ✓ Sterile surgical gloves
- ✓ Infusers, extenders, 3-way and high-pressure valves
- ✓ Suction probe, closed suction system
- ✓ Urine bag
- ✓ Breathing circuit, electrostatic filters
- ✓ Surgical brushes with betadine
- ✓ Hemostatic valves and Y-valves
- ✓ High-pressure connection in various lengths (90 cm, 50 cm, 30 cm, 15 cm)

The DM valuation is based on the 2018 call for tenders and the 2019 consultations.

➢ **Biological analysis**

Biological analyses were estimated by code.

These are B units converted into dinars, belonging to the Tunisian hospital nomenclature.

29

One B unit corresponds to 0.160 DT.

The list of biological analyses and their B units converted into dinars was provided by the patient management office (**tableIII**).

**Table IIIList of biological tests and their corresponding B units.**

| Biochemical analysis | B units |
|---|---|
| Ionogram | B100 |
| Creatinine | B 15 |
| Urea | B 15 |
| Blood glucose | B 15 |
| CRP | B 80 |
| Calcium | B 25 |
| Blood gases | B 120 |
| ASAT/ALAT | B 25 / B 25 |
| Total bilirubin / Direct bilirubin | B 15 / B 15 |
| Procalcitonin | B 200 |
| **Hematological analysis** | **B units** |
| NFS | B 60 |
| TP | B 20 |
| Blood grouping | B 30 |
| **Microbiological analysis** | **B units** |
| Protected tracheal sampling | B 80 |
| ECBU | B 70 |
| Therapeutic follow-up | B 200 |
| Antibiogram | B 80 |

*Pharmacological therapeutic monitoring of vancomycin.

> ➤ **Medical imaging and functional explorations:**

The main exploratory acts performed were:

- ✓ Cerebral, thoracic and abdominal computed tomography (CT).

✓ Magnetic resonance imaging (MRI).

✓ Electrocardiogram (ECG).

✓ Angioscanner.

They are accounted for according to the Tunisian hospital nomenclature by a code that is converted into dinars.

The codes are as follows:

✓ One Z unit (for brain, thoracic and abdominal CT scans) corresponds to 0.900 DT.

✓ One Ke unit (for ultrasound) corresponds to 1,200DT.

✓ One S unit (for scanners) corresponds to 9,000 DT.

✓ One I unit (for MRI) corresponds to 18,000 DT.

The list of medical imaging and functional explorations and their unit prices was provided to us by the patient management office (**tableIV**).

**Table IVList of medical imaging and functional explorations and their units**

| Exploratory acts | Units |
| --- | --- |
| Brain scan | S 10 |
| Chest CT | Z 25 |
| Abdominal scan | S 20 |
| MRI | I 15 |
| Angioscanner | S 35 |
| ECG | K 6 |

❖ **Direct non-medical costs**

Direct non-medical costs correspond to non-medical expenses incurred by the patient for the treatment of his illness[...47].

Direct non-medical costs are represented by:

➢ **Depreciation and amortization:**

- Depreciation of the embolization room costs 1,250 dinars per patient. This amount is used in the formula to calculate the total cost for each patient treated for an NRI procedure.
- The depreciation of care units is already included in hospital charges.

These financial data have been provided by INN's finance department.

> **Transportation costs:**

Transport costs were estimated and used in the formula to calculate the total cost for each patient treated for an NRI procedure.

There are two types of transport:

- **Public transport:**

Given the impossibility of determining the exact transport costs per patient, we have estimated these costs by region according to the tariffs allocated by the Ministry of Transport as of July 01, 2018 (**table V**).

**Table VList of tariffs awarded by the Ministry of Transport**

| Line | Rate in Dinars |
| --- | --- |
| Tunis - Béja | 7,600 |
| Tunis - Bizerte | 5,100 |
| Tunis - Gabès | 24,800 |
| Tunis - Grombalia | 2,750 |
| Tunis - Hammamet | 5,300 |
| Tunis - Jendouba | 11,200 |
| Tunis - Médenine | 29,550 |
| Tunis - Sfax | 17,400 |
| Tunis - Sidi Bouzid | 18,550 |
| Tunis - Sousse | 10,350 |

- **Medical transport**

Patients in critical condition were taken to INN by ambulance.

There are two types of ambulance:

- ✓ Ambulance from clinics, with fees set at 300 dinars.
- ✓ Ambulance from other hospitals and health centers, for which the fee is set at 50 dinars.

> **Unit loads**

Given that there is no recent cost accounting on the activity of the care units or on the indirect expenses of the INN, we have used the hospitalization costs which include the direct and indirect expenses of the care unit.

## 2.3.2.2. Indirect costs

Indirect costs are the value of production lost to society due to absence from work, disability and death. It is the loss of earnings due to the failure to produce what should have been produced. Since indirect costs do not directly influence expenditure on disease treatment, they are not easily measurable[49].

Three types of indirect costs can be distinguished [ .47

- Costs relating to the time spent on treatment by the patient, his or her family or friends.
- Costs associated with the patient's partial or total inability to work, or even his or her inability to enjoy leisure activities as a result of treatment.
- Loss of economic productivity following the patient's death.

The data required to assess indirect costs, i.e. absenteeism, were collected through direct interviews with patients in work-related occupations (**Appendix 1**).

## 2.3.2.3. Intangible costs

Intangible costs relate to the patient's suffering and psychosocial state.

They are linked to stress, anxiety, pain, and in general to all the losses of well-being and quality of life suffered by the patient[50].

This involves valuing the psychological harm or alteration in quality of life suffered by the patient or his family[50].

All these costs are real but rarely taken into account because of the extreme difficulty of their economic valuation, given their essentially qualitative and subjective nature[...50].

In our study, it was not possible to follow up patients after discharge from NIN, so intangible costs were not included.

## 2.4. Statistical analysis

The data from this study were analyzed using SPSS version 25 software .

### 2.4.1. Descriptive study

- **For categorical variables:**We calculated absolute and relative frequencies.
- **For quantitative variables**: We have calculated:
  - Means and standard deviations for variables following a normal distribution.
  - Medians and upper and lower quartiles for variables that do not follow a normal distribution.

### 2.4.2. Analytical study

- **Categorical variables:**The Mann Whitney U test was used for variables that do not follow a normal distribution.
- **Quantitative variables:**
  - ✓ Pearson's correlation coefficient was used for variables following a normal distribution.
  - ✓ Spearman's rank correlation coefficient was used for variables

that do not follow a normal distribution.

The relationship between two parameters was considered statistically significant when the P-value was less than 0.05.

If the result was statistically significant, the P-value and correlation coefficient were noted. The closer the correlation coefficient is to 1, the stronger the relationship between the two parameters.

Otherwise, for statistically insignificant results, only the P-value is noted.

## 2.5. Bibliographic research

We have carried out our bibliographical research in the following databases:

- PubMed (http://www.ncbi.nlm.nih.gov/pubmed)

- Science direct (http://www.sciencedirect.com)

- Elsevier Masson Consulte (http://www.em-consulte.com)

- Google scholar (http://www.scholar.google.com)

- New England Journal of medicine (https://www.nejm.org/)

- American Journal of Neuroradiology (http://www.ajnr.org/)

- French Neuroradiology Society (https://www.sfnr.net/)

The keywords used in the literature search were as follows:

- Interventional neuroradiology

- Embolization

- Catheterization and endovascular access

- Aneurysms

- Embolic agents (nBCA, onyx)

- Coils

- Arteriovenous malformations

- Dural arteriovenous fistulas

- Thrombectomy

- Pharmacoeconomics
- Cost analysis

Only studies in French or English were considered.

Zotero® was used to manage bibliographic references in the Vancouver style.

# 3. RESULTS

## 3.1. Description of the study population

The total number of patients who underwent embolization from March 19, 2019 to June 19, 2019 was 40, including:

- 29 patients underwent aneurysm embolization
- Patient embolized for ischemic stroke
- Two patients underwent embolization for an AVFd
- Five patients underwent embolization for an AVM
- Three patients underwent embolization for a tumor

The distribution of patients by diagnosis is shown in **Figure16**.

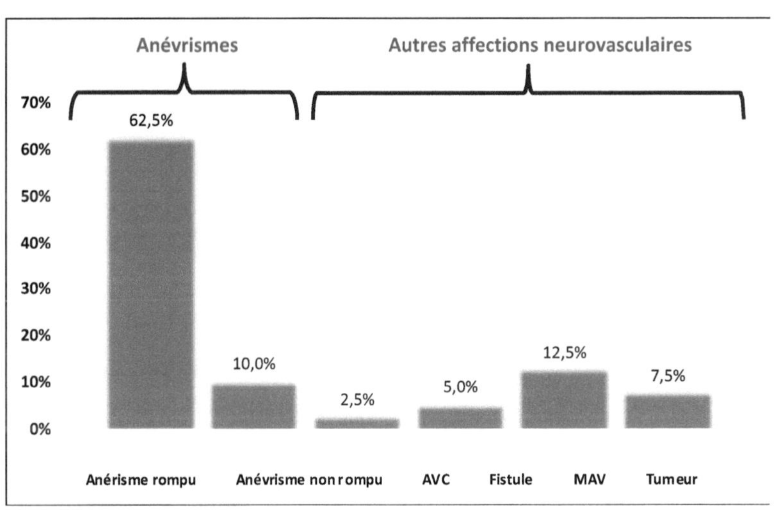


**Figure 16Distribution of patients by diagnosis**

## 3.1.1. Gender

The study population was made up of 50% men and 50% women, with a M/F sex ratio equal to one.

### 3.1.2. Age

The median age of the study population was 54, with a minimum of four years and a maximum of 80.

The age distribution of patients is shown in **figure17.**

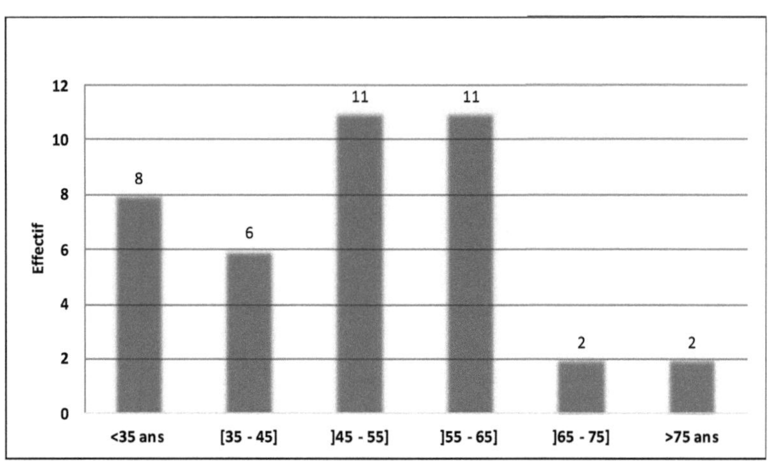


**Figure 17Patient distribution by age group**

### 3.1.3. Socioeconomic level and professional activity

The majority of our study population (n=32) was non-active, i.e. retired, housewife, student and unemployed. The remaining eight patients had a professional activity.

The distribution of patients according to their state of professional activity is shown in **figure 18.**

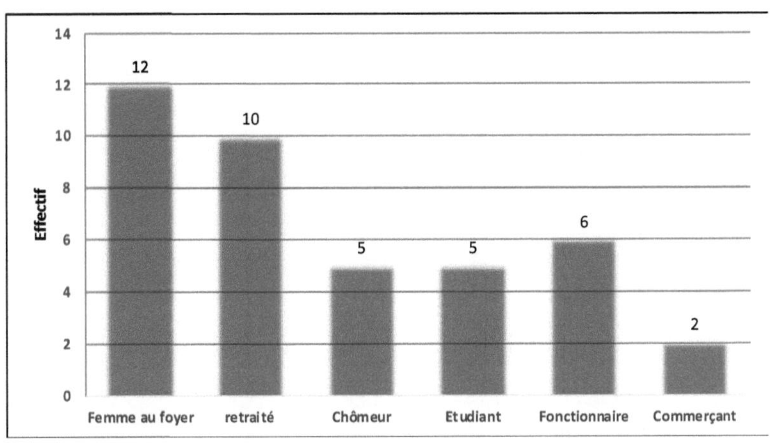


**Figure 18Distribution of patients by professional activity**

## 3.1.4. Length of hospital stay

The median length of hospital stay for all patients was four and a half days, with extremes ranging from one to 30 days.

## 3.1.5. Cardiovascular risk factors

Twenty-two of the 40 patients in our study had risk factors.

The distribution of patients according to associated risk factors is shown in **Figure 19.**

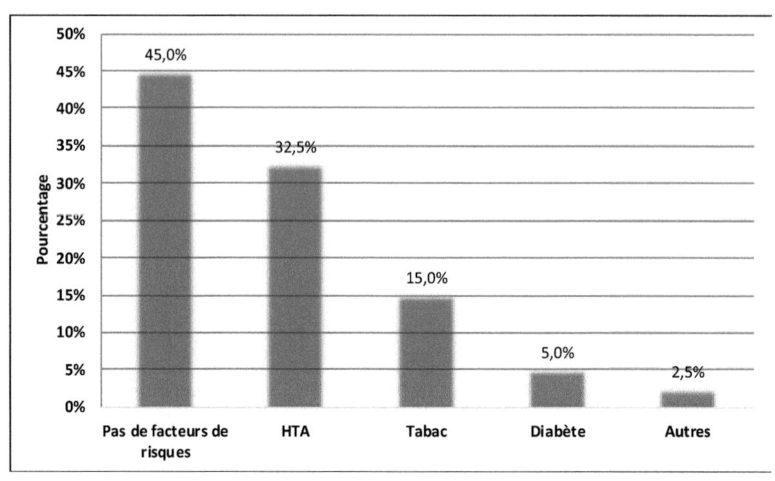


**Figure 19Distribution of patients according to risk factors**

## 3.1.6 Evolution

For a total of 40 patients who underwent embolization, six patients (15%) presented a post embolization complication, five of whom (12.5%) died. These complications are divided into:

Procedural complications:

- Ischemic stroke following aneurysm occlusion (n=1)
- Aneurysm rupture with cerebral hemorrhage and coma (n=1)

Complications unrelated to the procedure:

- Nosocomial infections (n=2).
- Cardiorespiratory arrest (n=1).
- Hydrocephalus associated with thrombophlebitis and respiratory distress (n=1).

Patient outcomes and complications following embolization are shown in **Figure 20.**

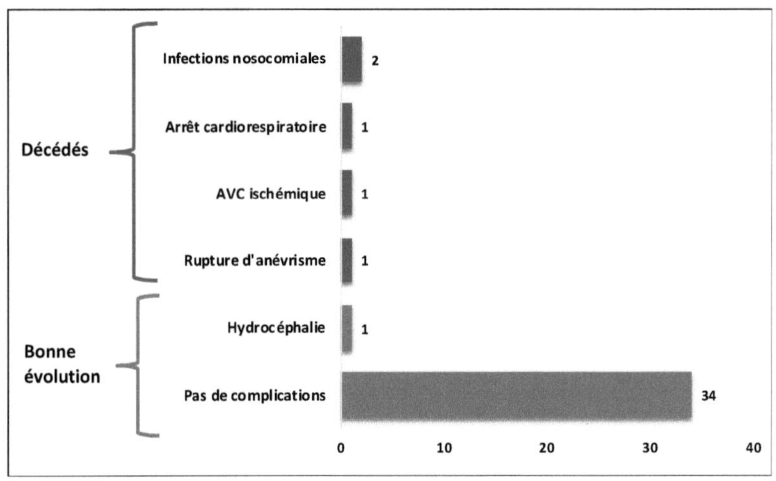



**Figure 20Evolution of patients and the complications they presented post-embolization**

## 3.2. Clinical results and descriptive analyses by procedure

### 3.2.1. Management of aneurysms

A description of the clinical parameters of patients treated with aneurysm embolization in our study is presented in **Table VI**.

A total of 29 aneurysms were treated, of which 13 were men (44.8%) and 16 (55.2%) women. The mean age of the patients was 53.9 plus or minus 13.9 years.

**Table VI:Clinical parameters of patients treated with aneurysm embolization**

| Patient characteristics | Number |
| --- | --- |
| **Gender** | |
| Men | 13 (44,8%) |
| Woman | 16 (55,2%) |
| **Age** | |
| Median (min - max) | 55 (17 - 80) |
| **Total length of stay** | |
| Median (min - max) | 5 (1 - 20) |
| **Comorbidities** | |
| Hypertension | 11 (37,9%) |
| Tobacco | 5 (17,2%) |
| Diabetes | 1 (3,4%) |
| **Qualifying the aneurysm** | |
| Broken | 25 (86,2%) |
| Unbroken | 4 (13,8%) |
| **Aneurysm size** | |
| 0 - 5 mm | 14 (48 ,3%) |
| 6 - 10 mm | 11 (37,9%) |
| 11 - 15 mm | 4 (13,8%) |
| **Aneurysm collar** | |
| Narrow | 25 (82,8%) |
| Large | 4 (17,2%) |
| **Aneurysm location** | |
| Previous communicant | 13 (44,8%) |
| Carotid | 8 (27,6%) |
| Vertebrobasilar artery | 3 (10,3%) |
| Other locations | 5 (17,2%) |
| **Complications** | |
| Yes | 5 (17,2%) |
| No | 24 (82,8%) |
| **Evolution** | |
| Good | 24 (82,8%) |
| Deaths | 5 (17,2%) |

### 3.2.2. Management of other neurovascular disorders

### 3.2.2.1. Arteriovenous malformations

A total of five AVMs were treated. The median age of the patients was 24 years, with extremes ranging from four to 41 years. The median overall stay was three days, with extremes ranging from two to 30 days, and only one patient was admitted to the intensive care unit for six days. This same patient presented a complication with a favorable outcome. There were no deaths in this group.

### 3.2.2.2. Spinal dural fistula

A total of two fistulas were treated. The median overall stay in the medical units was three and a half days. There were no complications or deaths.

### 3.2.2.3. Tumor

A total of three tumors were treated by embolization. The median overall stay in the medical units was two days. There were no complications or deaths.

### 3.2.2.4. Cerebrovascular accident

A single 55-year-old male patient was treated by thrombectomy for ischemic stroke localized to the left internal carotid artery. Overall stay in the neurology department was 11 days. The patient progressed well and there were no complications.

A description of the study population and clinical parameters according to the neurovascular pathology treated by embolization, is presented in **Table VII**.

**Table VIICharacteristics of the study population and clinical outcomes**

| Neurovascular disorders | | Aneurysm | MAV | Fistula | Tumor | AVC |
|---|---|---|---|---|---|---|
| Number | | 29 | 5 | 2 | 3 | 1 |
| Gender | Men | 13 | 3 | 1 | 2 | 1 |
| | Woman | 16 | 2 | 1 | 1 | 0 |
| Average age (years) | | 53,9 | 24,8 | 61,5 | 35,5 | 55 |
| Median overall length of stay | | 5 | 3 | 3,5 | 2 | 11 |
| Complications | | Yes | Yes | Yes | No | No |
| Evolution | Deaths | 5 | 0 | 0 | 0 | 0 |
| | Good | 24 | 5 | 2 | 3 | 1 |

## 3.3. Cost analysis

### 3.3.1. Analysis of total direct costs

The median of total direct costs in the study population was 14,046 DT, with a minimum of 7,079 DT and a maximum of 36,325 DT. The mean was 14,942 DT with a standard deviation of 5,653 DT.

The distribution of these costs in the population is shown in **figure 21.**

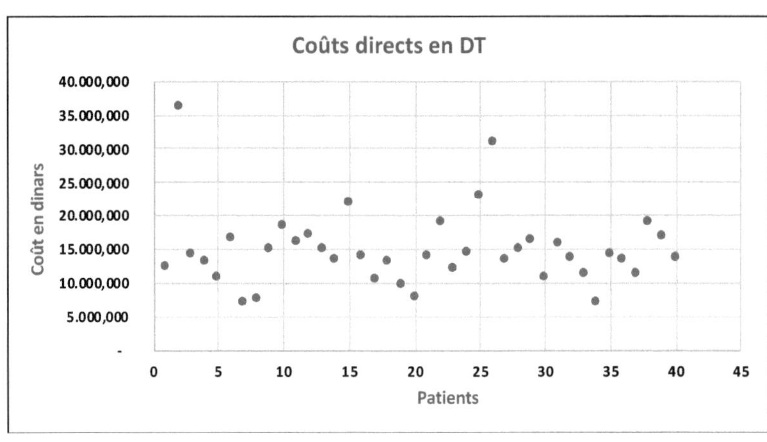


**Figure 21Distribution of total direct costs per patient in dinars in the population**

The majority of total direct costs per patient (77.5%) were in the range from 10,000 to 20,000 DT.

The **figure 22**shows the breakdown of total direct patient costs by cost category.

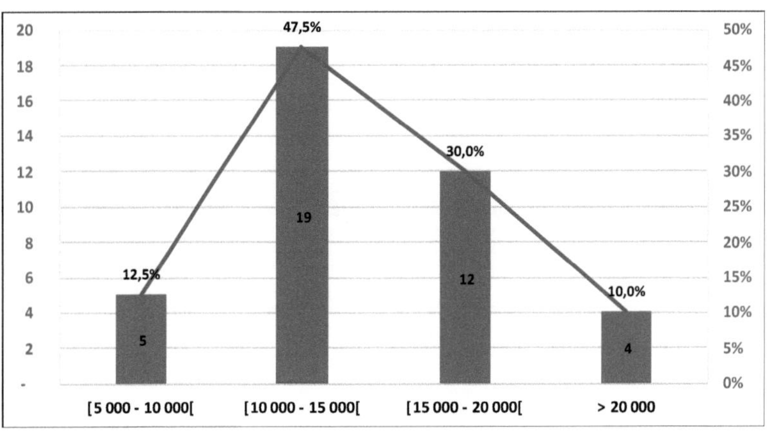



**Figure 22Breakdown of total direct patient costs by cost category
in dinars**

The analysis of total direct costs per patient by diagnosis is shown in **table VIII.**

**Table VIIIAnalysis of total direct costs per patient by diagnosis.**

| Neurovascular disorders | | Number | Median costs (DT) | Average costs (DT) | Minimum (DT) | Maximum (DT) |
|---|---|---|---|---|---|---|
| **Aneurysm** | **Broken** | 29 | 14 244 | 15 031 | 8 005 | 36 325 |
| | | 25 | 14 244 | 16 877 | | |
| | **Unbroken** | 4 | 14 271 | 14 915 | | |
| **MAV** | | 5 | 13 656 | 13 021 | 7 746 | 18 439 |
| **Tumor** | | 3 | 15 148 | 14 906 | 13 616 | 15 954 |
| **Fistula** | | 2 | 7 136 | 7 136 | 7 079 | 7 192 |

| AVC | 1 | 13 138 | - | - | - |

### 3.3.2. Direct medical costs

The median direct medical costs per patient were 12,746 DT, with a minimum of 5,829 DT and a maximum of 35,025 DT. The mean was 13,658 DT ± 5,654 DT.

The distribution of direct medical costs in the population is shown in **table IX.**

**Table IXDistribution of direct medical costs in the population.**

| Parameters | Median costs (DT) | Average (DT) | Minimum (DT) | Maximum (DT) | Percentage of average cost |
|---|---|---|---|---|---|
| Medicines | 335 | 487 | 216 | 1 936 | 3,6% |
| Medical devices | 11 774 | 12 593 | 4 825 | 33 982 | 92,2% |
| Biological analysis | 44,500 | 111 | 44,500 | 474 | 0,8% |
| X-ray examinations | 30 | 75 | 30 | 435 | 0,5% |
| Hospitalization costs | 180 | 233 | 40 | 1 280 | 1,7% |
| Medical and paramedical staff costs | 159 | 159 | - | - | 1.2% |
| Direct medical costs | 12 746 | 13 658 | 5 829 | 35 025 | 100% |

Pharmaceuticals account for 95.8% of the median direct cost, with 92.2% for medical devices.

The breakdown of total costs by diagnosis is shown in the **table** below. Xand the share (in%) of the cost of pharmaceutical products (drugs and DM) in the total average cost is shown in **figure23**.

**Table XBreakdown of total costs by diagnosis**

| Parameters | Total cost aneurysm | Total cost MAV | Total cost FAVd | Total tumor cost | Total cost Stroke |
|---|---|---|---|---|---|
| **Pharmaceutical products** | 85,4% | 84,7% | 76,8% | 89,2% | 82,4% |
| **Amortization of NRI room** | 9% | 10% | 18% | 8,5% | 9,4% |
| **Hospital stay** | 1,4% | 2,7% | 1,9% | 0,5% | 2,9% |
| **Other** | 4,2% | 2,6% | 3,3% | 1,8% | 5,3% |

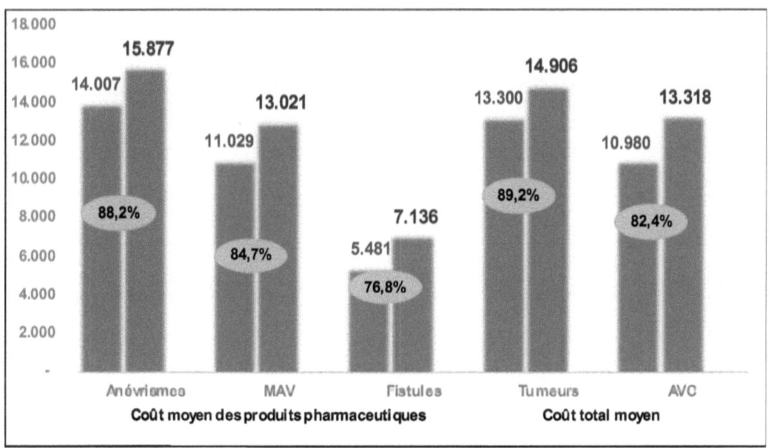


**Figure 23Average cost of pharmaceutical products by diagnosis in the population**

Spearman's non-parametric Rho correlation gave us a statistically significant result at the 0.01 level (p <0.01) concerning the relationship between pharmaceutical costs and direct medical costs with the following correlation coefficients:

- The drugs had a P value = 0.002 with a correlation coefficient equal to 0.45.
- Medical devices had a p-value = 0.001 with a high correlation coefficient equal to 0.96.

Expenditure on drugs and medical devices can be broken down into two categories: firstly, pharmaceutical products used during the operation, and secondly, those used during hospitalization. **TableXI**provides a summary of these costs.

**Table XICosts of drugs and medical devices during the operation and during hospitalization.**

| | During the intervention | | During hospitalization | |
|---|---|---|---|---|
| Cost in dinars | Medicines | Medical devices | Medicines | Medical devices |
| **Median** | 288 | 11 773 | 26 | 1 |
| **Average** | 386 | 12 585 | 101 | 8 |
| **Maximum** | 1 100 | 33 979 | 1 715 | 100 |
| **Minimum** | 189 | 4 823 | 2 | 1 |
| **Percentage of direct medical costs** | 2.8% | 92% | 0.8% | 0.06% |

The cost of medical devices used during the procedure accounted for the bulk of direct medical costs (92%). The cost of those used during hospitalization was considered negligible, accounting for only 0.06% of direct medical costs.

### 3.3.2.1. Cost of medical devices

The results for medical device costs by neurovascular condition are summarized in **tablesXII, XIII, XIV**and**XV**.

**Table XIICosts of medical devices used during aneurysm embolization of aneurysms without Remodeling technique.**

| Number of patients | 22 | | |
|---|---|---|---|
| Designation | Average cost (DT) | Percentage of average DM costs | Percentage of total average cost |
| Coils | 9 351 | 69,5% | 59,2% |
| Microguides | 1 245 | 9,3% | 7,9% |
| Microcatheters | 1 468 | 10,9% | 9,3% |
| Carrier catheters | 797 | 5,9% | 5% |
| Other | 581 | 4,3% | 3,7% |
| Average DM cost | 13 452 | 99,9% | - |
| Average total cost | 15 800 | - | 85,1% |

*DM used during the procedure, such as guidewires, hemostatic valves, injection syringes, sterile drapes, etc.

**Table XIIICosts of medical devices used during aneurysm embolization with the Remodeling technique.**

| Number of patients | 7 | | |
|---|---|---|---|
| Designation | Average cost (DT) | Percentage of average DM costs | Percentage of total average cost |
| Coils | 6 501 | 46,9% | 40,3% |
| Balloon | 2 993 | 21,6% | 18,6% |
| Microguides | 1 246 | 9% | 7,8% |
| Microcatheters | 1 746 | 12,6% | 10,8% |
| Carrier catheters | 797 | 5,8% | 4,9% |
| Other | 565 | 4% | 3,5% |
| Average DM cost | 13 850 | 99,9% | - |
| Average total cost | 16 118 | - | 85,9% |

*DM used during the procedure, such as guidewires, haemostatic valves, injection syringes, sterile drapes, etc.

**Table XIVCosts of medical devices used during embolization of AVMs and tumors**

| Number of patients | | 8 | |
|---|---|---|---|
| Designation | Average cost (DT) | Percentage of total DM costs | Percentage of total average cost |
| Surgical adhesives | 2 956 | 26,2% | 21,5% |
| Microguides | 1 619 | 14,3% | 11,8% |
| Microcatheters | 5 388 | 47,7% | 39,2% |
| Carrier catheters | 797 | 7,1% | 5,8% |
| Other | 520 | 4,6% | 3,8% |
| Average DM cost | 11 288 | 99,9% | - |
| Average total cost | 13 728 | - | 82,2% |

*DM used during the procedure, such as guidewires, hemostatic valves, injection syringes, sterile drapes, etc.

**Table XVCosts of medical devices used during AVF embolizationd**

| Number of patients | | 2 | |
|---|---|---|---|
| Designation | Average cost (DT) | Percentage of total DM costs | Percentage of total average cost |
| Surgical adhesives | 375 | 7,7% | 6,4% |
| Microguides | 1 855 | 38% | 31,7% |
| Microcatheters | 2 200 | 45% | 37,6% |
| Carrier catheters | 79,5 | 1,6% | 1,4% |
| Other | 375 | 7,7% | 6,4% |
| Average DM cost | 4 886 | 91,9% | - |
| Average total cost | 7 136 | - | 63,2% |

*DM used during the procedure, such as guidewires, hemostatic valves, injection syringes, sterile drapes...

For aneurysm management, coils alone, for embolization without remodeling, and coils combined with balloons, for embolization with remodeling, accounted for the bulk of medical device costs.

On the other hand, in patients treated by embolization for AVMs or FAVd or tumors, microcatheters, microguides and embolic agents accounted for the largest share of medical device costs.

For ischemic stroke thrombectomy, DM accounted for 80.6% of the total average cost.

### 3.3.2.2. Drug costs

Drug costs represented the total expenditure on drugs used per patient during the operation and hospitalization.

Drugs accounted for 3.6% of direct medical costs, of which 2.8% were those used during the procedure.

**Table XVI** summarizes the cost of drugs used during the procedure, by therapeutic class: anesthetics, injectable anticoagulants, iodinated contrast media and others.

**Table XVI: Cost of drugs used in interventional neuroradiology procedures**

| Number of patients | | 40 |
|---|---|---|
| Designation | Average cost (DT) | Percentage of total drug costs |
| Anaesthetic drugs | 121 | 25% |
| Iodinated contrast media | 204 | 42% |
| Injectable anticoagulants | 8 | 1,6% |
| Calcium channel blockers (Nimodipine) | 31 | 6% |

| **Other** | 12 | 2,5% |

* Other drugs used on a case-by-case basis as required during the embolization procedure.

Iodinated contrast media (42%) and drugs used for general anesthesia (25%) accounted for the largest share of drug costs during the procedure. Drugs used during hospitalization accounted for only 0.8% of direct medical costs. Their cost was influenced mainly by length of stay and the occurrence of post-embolization complications.

- Pearson's bivariate correlation gave us a statistically significant result at the 0.01 level ($p = 0.001$) concerning the relationship between drug costs during hospitalization and length of hospital stay, with a correlation coefficient of 0.65.
- The Mann-Whitney rank-sum test yielded a statistically significant test with a value of $p = 0.009$ for the relationship between drug costs during hospitalization and the occurrence of complications.


### 3.3.3. Direct non-medical costs

The median direct non-medical cost was 1,285 DT, with a minimum of 1,250 DT and a maximum of 1,550 DT.

- Depreciation and amortization amounted to DT 1,250.
- The median cost of transport was 50 DT, with extremes ranging from 5 to 300 DT.

The evaluation of direct non-medical costs did not have a significant influence on total costs. Indeed, Spearman's non-parametric Rho correlation gave us a statistically insignificant result with a p-value $> 0.05$ ($p = 0.71$) concerning the relationship between direct non-medical costs and total cost.

### 3.3.4. Analysis of indirect costs

The evaluation of indirect costs, represented in our study by absenteeism, had little influence on the total cost. Only one patient out of forty benefited from a 9-day medical rest, raising the indirect cost to 180 dinars. Indeed, Spearman's non-parametric Rho correlation between indirect costs and total cost gave us a statistically insignificant result with a p-value $> 0.05$ $(p = 0.58)$.

The following reasons may explain this non-correlation:

- In the case of short-term absences, there is no loss of productivity as the work could be done by a colleague or the individual himself on his return.
- non-active patients accounted for a large proportion of the study population (80%).

### 3.3.5. Analysis of intangible costs

In our study, patient follow-up after discharge from NIN was not included, so intangible costs were not assessed.

### 3.3.6. Analysis of total hospital costs

The median total cost in the study population was 14,046 DT, with a minimum of 7,079 DT and a maximum of 36,325 DT.

Furthermore, the correlation between direct medical costs and total costs is significant at the 0.01 level $(p < 0.001)$, with a correlation coefficient of 1.

This correlation shows that total cost is entirely dependent on direct medical costs, and more specifically on spending on medical devices used during the procedure.

## 4. DISCUSSION

### 4.1. Conclusion of the study

In our study, we were mainly interested in determining the total cost of an interventional neuroradiology procedure. Secondly, to compare this total cost with the lump sums allocated by the Caisse Nationale d'Assurance Maladie. And finally, to identify the main parameters associated with variations in the total cost of this procedure.

Our work is the first Tunisian study to assess the cost of NRI. We were not only interested in evaluating the cost of endovascular treatment of aneurysms, but also that of AVMs, FAVd, tumors and ischemic strokes. In fact, for certain pathologies such as AVFd and tumors, few descriptive literature references or cost analyses were found.

According to our study, the total cost of embolization of a vascular malformation of the central nervous system varies from a minimum of 7,079 DT to a maximum of 36,325 DT, with a median of 14,046 DT.

For aneurysm embolization, the median total cost is 14,244 DT, with extremes ranging from 8,005 DT to 36,325 DT. For AVMs, the median cost is 13,656 DT, with a minimum of 7,746 DT and a maximum of 18,439 DT. For tumors, hospitalization costs range from 13,616 DT to 15,954 DT, with a median of 15,148 DT. For the treatment of fistulas and strokes, the median total costs are 7,136 DT and 13,138 DT respectively.

Our study reported that total cost is significantly influenced by the cost of pharmaceutical products, notably medical devices ($p<0.001$) and drugs ($p=0.02$).

Furthermore, for aneurysms, we have shown that the number of coils used ($p<0.001$), the number of microcatheters ($p<0.001$), the size ($p=0.021$) and the width of the neck ($p=0.048$) of the aneurysm have a significant influence on the total cost of the procedure.

As for AVMs, fistulas and tumors, the cost of their intervention is influenced by the quantity of embolic agents (p=0.003) and the number of microcatheters (p<0.001).

However, whether the aneurysm was ruptured or unruptured (p=0.81), the length of hospital stay (p=0.14) and cardiovascular risk factors (p=0.12) had no influence on the total cost of the procedure.

The reimbursement system for embolization of a neurovascular pathology in Tunisia consists, for patients affiliated to the CNAM, of full coverage by the insurance system.

The CNAM is initially offering the same fixed price of 7,000 DT for endovascular treatment of aneurysms, AVMs, FAVd and tumors. For thrombectomies of ischemic strokes, the package allocated is 12,000 DT. For patients on the full-fee plan, the NRI procedure and hospital stay are entirely at their own expense.

For indigent patients, they are paid for by the institute.

## 4.2. Management of aneurysms

Since the advent of endovascular techniques in the treatment of intracranial aneurysms, their therapeutic approach has changed considerably. Two major studies, ISAT [3for ruptured aneurysms, and ISUIA [4] for unruptured aneurysms. Following the publication of these two studies, the choice of treatment shifted from surgery to embolization.

### 4.2.1. Gender

Data in the literature show a predominance of women in the endovascular treatment of aneurysms, with sex ratios ranging from 0.38 to 0.93[51-54].

In our study, the sex ratio was 0.81, within the range reported in the literature.

## 4.2.2. Age

The median age in our series of endovascular treatment of aneurysms was 55 years (17 - 80 years). We found a homogeneous, age-independent distribution of patients with intracranial aneurysms.

In a French retrospective study by Labalette et al. the median age reported was 52 years, with extremes ranging from 26 to 84 years[54].

## 4.2.3. Length of stay, trends and cost of hospitalization

In our study, the median length of stay was five days, with a maximum of 20 days (corresponding to a prolonged hospital stay due to a post-operative complication of nosocomial infection) and a minimum of 24 hours (for post-embolization monitoring).

The Moroccan study by Cheikh et al. reported a median length of stay of seven days, one day in the intensive care unit and five days in the medical units, with a minimum of four days and a maximum of 11 days [55].

The French study by Labalette et al. found a median length of stay of five days, which coincides with our duration, with extremes ranging from two to 31 days[54].

Thromboembolic complications are probably the most common serious complication in interventional neuroradiology. The risk of thrombosis is linked to aggression on the vascular endothelium during catheterization maneuvers, to the contrast medium and embolization material used, and to catheters[56]. The main method of risk prevention is to maintain effective anticoagulation throughout the procedure with heparin [57]. Thromboembolic complications are generally less severe in AVMs than in aneurysms[58].

Vasospasm is the main complication of subarachnoid hemorrhage (SAH), potentially leading to death and serious neurological complications. Early vasospasm is a reduction in vascular caliber immediately after SAH and up to three to four hours later. Late vasospasm, most often beginning 4$^{\text{ème}}$ days after SAH, with a peak around 7$^{\text{ème}}$ days, can occur near or far from the ruptured aneurysm[48]. Treatment of this complication is mainly based on chemical angioplasty, involving intra-arterial injection of a vasodilator such as nimodipine (Nimotop®)[48].

Another frequent complication of aneurysm embolization is bleeding. The risk of aneurysmal rupture during endovascular treatment is 2.5%[59]. Diagnosis is made by contrast injection, which immediately confirms extravascular leakage or, on the contrary, eliminates the hypothesis of rupture. The immediate course of action involves reversing the effect of heparin with protamine sulfate at a dose of 1 mg per 100 U of UFH. Filling of the aneurysm sac should be continued in order to occlude the aneurysm as quickly as possible and stop the bleeding[60].

In the literature, we find morbidity percentages ranging from eight to 29% and mortality from four to 5.7% of the study population[51,52,61]. Ischemic stroke and aneurysmal rupture were the two most frequent complications reported in the Pakistani study by Zubair Tahir et al. which aimed to assess the cost-effectiveness of clipping versus coiling of intracranial aneurysms after subarachnoid hemorrhage[52].

In our study, complications occurred in 17.2% (n=5) of patients treated by aneurysm embolization, with the majority not related to the endovascular procedure but rather to postoperative hospitalization. The mortality rate associated with these complications was 100%. All five patients died as a result of nosocomial infections, ischemic stroke following aneurysm occlusion, subarachnoid hemorrhage due to aneurysm rupture, and cardiorespiratory arrest.

On the other hand, we were also interested in determining the determinants of hospitalization costs, and we reported that the overall cost was not influenced by the total length of stay (p=0.14) or hospitalization in the intensive care unit (p=0.12), which can be explained by the low cost of pharmaceutical products used during hospitalization and the low cost of the hospital stay itself.

The Moroccan study by Cheikh et al. reported the same results as ours and showed that there was no correlation between, on the one hand, the total length of hospital stay or only the intensive care stay and, on the other hand, the overall cost (p=0.096) and (p=0.073)[53].

However, in a retrospective Canadian study by Bekelis et al. aimed at developing and validating a predictive model of the cost of hospitalization after coiling of a cerebral aneurysm, the impact of hospital stay on the overall cost of care was shown with a value of p<0.0001[51].

This study showed that the initial cost of hospitalization was a major component of the overall economic burden of healthcare, and that one of the main factors in the variation of this cost was the length of hospitalization[51].

Another French retrospective study by Labalette et al., whose aim was to assess the hospital cost of cerebral aneurysm embolization and compare it with the revenue generated by the reimbursement system, also reported the significant share of the cost of the hospital stay in the overall charge, which represented 42% of the overall cost (€6,908 for €16,356)[54].

This difference in the cost of a hospital stay and the impact of length of stay on the overall economic burden can be explained by the fact that it is difficult to transpose our economic estimates to medical and economic studies carried out in other countries, given the differences in the organization of the medical care system and in the pricing structure.

### 4.2.4. Cardiovascular risk factors

In our study, we demonstrated that 37.9% (11) of patients were hypertensive, 17.2% (5) smokers and 3.4% (1) diabetics.

The retrospective study by Elewa et al. which aimed to discuss the technical and management results of the first series of symptomatic and asymptomatic cerebral saccular aneurysm cases treated by embolization in Egypt, reported 41.9% of subjects who were hypertensive, 38.7% smokers and 12.9% diabetics [61].

Another retrospective Canadian study by Bekelis et al. also found a majority of hypertensive patients (55.5%), followed by 36.8% of smokers[51].

Although hypertension and smoking are considered risk factors for haemorrhagic stroke, they do not appear to influence the overall cost (p=0.12). The Moroccan study by Cheikh et al. reported the same result, with a p-value equal to 0.77[53].

### 4.2.5. Total cost and influencing factors

According to our study, the total cost of an endovascular procedure on an intracranial aneurysm varies from a minimum of 8,005 DT to a maximum of 36,325 DT, with an average of 15,887 DT per patient. The total cost of 11 patients was above the average, and the 29 patients treated had a hospitalization cost in excess of 7,000 DT, being the initial package reimbursed by CNAM to cover all embolization costs.

The average cost of endovascular treatment in France was estimated in the retrospective study by Labalette et al. at €16,356 (TD 29,441) (45).

In Morocco, the study by Cheikh et al. reported an average cost of €7,528 (16,562 DT), with extremes ranging from €4,784 (10,525 DT) to €32,172 (70,778 DT) (44).

In our study, we have shown that the cost of pharmaceutical products accounts for the bulk of total costs, with a percentage of 85.4%, followed by depreciation of the neuroradiology room (9%), the hospital stay (1.4%) and other costs representing 4.2% of total hospitalization costs.

In our study, we were interested in separating the cost of pharmaceutical products between those used during the procedure and those used during hospitalization, and found that drugs and DM used during the procedure represent 94.8% of direct medical costs, with a cost of 12,061 DT, while the share of those used during hospitalization is negligible (0.86%).

There was a statistically significant correlation between the cost of pharmaceuticals and the number of coils and other medical devices used (p<0.001). It is also significant between the cost of pharmaceuticals (medical devices) and aneurysm size (p=0.021) and neck size (p=0.048) respectively. These results are consistent in that, as aneurysm size increases, so does the number of coils required to fill the bag.

Furthermore, the number of devices used varies according to the size of the neck. This can be explained by the fact that when the size of the neck exceeds a certain value, the neuroradiologist is obliged to resort to the Remodeling technique, using either a balloon or a stent for greater safety during filling of the aneurysm sac, which implies a significant increase in the costs incurred.

Our study also showed that among the DM used during the procedure, coils accounted for the bulk of the total cost, regardless of the technique used (without or with Remodeling), with costs of 9,351 and 6,501 DT respectively, followed by balloons for the Remodeling technique with a cost of 2,993 DT, microcatheters and microguides in almost equal proportions with a cost of 1,246 and 1,746 DT, followed by the carrier catheter with a cost of 797 DT, then other DM with a cost of 581 DT.

In the French study, which aimed to assess the hospital cost of cerebral aneurysm embolization, Labalette et al. also looked at the cost of DM used during the endovascular procedure and reported an average cost of €5,226 (7,160 DT) for ruptured aneurysms and €7,746 (10,611 DT) for unruptured ones, with 55.7% represented by the cost of coils[54].

Another study conducted by Zubair Tahir et al. in Pakistan aimed to compare clinical outcomes, resource consumption and cost-effectiveness of endovascular treatment versus surgical clipping in a developing country. This study also determined the DM cost, which amounted to $3,000 (4,110 DT), representing 59.2% of the average total hospitalization cost[52].

In another retrospective American study carried out at the University of Utah by Twitchell et al., the aim of which was to assess the specific cost drivers for surgical clipping and coilingendovascularization of ruptured and unruptured intracranial aneurysms, the cost of pharmaceuticals used during the embolization procedure accounted for 50.8% of the total cost, including 43.2% for DM[62].

These results also coincide with our study, in which the cost of pharmaceutical products, particularly DM, accounts for the bulk of the total cost of hospitalization.


### 4.2.6. Aneurysm embolization and pharmaco-economics

The ISAT trial demonstrated that endovascular treatment gave better clinical results, measured at 2 months and 1 year of follow-up, for aneurysms suitable for both coilingendovascular and neurosurgical clipping [3]. Aneurysm embolization is increasingly used worldwide, even in developing countries. In the USA, the rate of endovascular treatment rose between 2002 and 2008 from 30% to 63% for unruptured aneurysms, and from 17% to 58% for ruptured aneurysms[63].

Against this backdrop, a number of studies have assessed the cost-effectiveness of coilingendovascularization versus surgical clipping of ruptured or unruptured intracranial aneurysms, and compared clinical outcomes.

In a Pakistani study, Zubair Tahir et al. evaluated the cost-effectiveness of clipping versus coiling of intracranial aneurysms after subarachnoid hemorrhage in a developing country[52].

The cost of coiling was 62% higher than that of clipping, without the added benefit of reduced morbidity. Hospitalization costs were lower in the endovascular group, due to the shorter length of stay compared with the surgical group. However, the benefits of this apparent reduction in length of stay were offset by the higher price of the endovascular procedure and the cost of pharmaceuticals. The average cost of endovascular treatment was estimated at $5,070 (6,946 DT) in Pakistan[52].

Ballet et al presented an opposite conclusion in a retrospective study carried out in France. They concluded that while the endovascular procedure tended to be more costly in terms of sterile single-use medical devices (coils, microcatheters.), this increase was more than offset by savings on personnel costs, as well as on the duration and cost of hospitalization[64].

The endovascular technique allows for a shorter hospital stay, patients tend to return to normal activity more quickly and have a favorable functional outcome compared to patients who have undergone neurosurgical intervention[64].

A retrospective study in the United States by Lad et al. aimed to determine the long-term economic impact of coilingendovascularization versus surgical clipping for the treatment of intracranial aneurysms; the total cost for patients who underwent coiling was $82,986 (132,777DT)[65].

As the financing system is totally different from ours, American studies on the cost of embolization cannot be transposed to Tunisia.

In this study, they found that although clipping was associated with more complications, it resulted in fewer reinterventions, so that the cost of clipping and coiling was comparable at five years. In contrast, patients in the endovascular group accumulated more costs due to longer follow-up due to high rates of reinterventions and angiograms[65].

In this sense, several studies have looked at the treatment of aneurysms and have reported that the retreatment rate is much higher in patients who have undergone coilingendovascularization and this can be explained by a recanalization rate, or the return of blood flow to the aneurysm, which is higher when aneurysms are treated by embolization[3,66,67].

In our case, the first follow-up angiogram is performed 6 months after aneurysm embolization, with the possibility of endovascular reintervention followed by further angiograms.

The endovascular technique offers many advantages for patients, but cannot be successful in all types of intracranial aneurysm. Both surgical and endovascular techniques remain indispensable for the treatment of aneurysms[3].


### 4.3. Management of other neurovascular disorders

In our study, we reported five cases of AVM, with a median age of 24 years, ranging from four to 41 years, and a majority of males. The median length of stay was three days, with extremes ranging from two to 30 days (corresponding to admission to the intensive care unit and then to neuropediatrics following a post-operative complication such as hydrocephalus).

The study conducted in the USA by Rutledge et al. on the determinants of the cost of management of arteriovenous malformations, reported for the study group of preoperative embolization, an average age of $38 \pm 17$ years with a female majority with 65% women for 45% men on a sample larger than ours including 49 Patients[68].

In our study, we evaluated the median overall cost of an endovascular procedure on an AVM, which amounted to 13,656 DT, with a minimum of 7,746 and a maximum of 18,439 DT.

Total obliteration of AVMs is often not achieved from the very first procedure, requiring several embolization courses or a combination of different disciplines including interventional neuroradiology, surgery and radiotherapy to achieve total occlusion of the AVM[5].

The median overall cost reported by the Scottish *IntracranialVascular Malformation Study* by Miller et al. was £16,938, equivalent to 37,264 Tunisian Dinars. They determined the direct healthcare costs and estimated the indirect cost of lost productivity for the entire study population[69].

In the American study by Rutledge et al, surgery with preoperative embolization was the most expensive procedure, with a mean cost of $91,948, with a minimum of $79,914 and a maximum of $140,600[68].

On the other hand, while preoperative embolization followed by surgery is the most costly treatment, reducing the number and duration of interventions can make it the most cost-effective treatment[68].

Our study shows that for the endovascular treatment of tumors and FAVd, the overall median cost of each pathology was 15,148 DT and 7,136 DT respectively. Determination of the factors influencing variation in the median cost of AVMs showed that the cost of pharmaceuticals accounted for more than half of the overall median cost.

The median overall cost of these three conditions is directly dependent on the pharmaceuticals, notably microcatheters (p<0.001) and embolic agents (p=0.003), used during the procedure.

Whatever the neurovascular pathology to be treated endovascularly, the cost of DM used during the procedure accounts for over 60% of the total average cost. This may be explained by the need to change microcatheters during the procedure, due to precipitation of the embolic agent in the catheter lumen.

To date, there are few data on the cost of endovascular treatment of cerebral AVMs, tumors and FAVd.

As regards thrombectomy for ischemic stroke, we reported a single case with a cost of 13,138 DT, 80.6% of which was accounted for by the cost of DM.

A UK study estimated the average total cost of mechanical thrombectomy and subsequent hospital care in the first 24 hours at 39,045 DT. The main cost driver was the pharmaceuticals used during the thrombectomy procedure, which accounted for 73% of the total cost[70].

Recent clinical trials have demonstrated the efficacy of mechanical thrombectomy in acute ischemic stroke. In 2015, the European Stroke Organization (ESO) updated recommendations for the treatment of acute ischemic stroke to advocate the use of mechanical thrombectomy[71].


## 4.4. Weaknesses of our study

This is a prospective study in which the calculation of hospitalization costs included direct costs and indirect costs represented solely by the patient's loss of professional productivity for the duration of his or her hospitalization. The follow-up of the patient after discharge from hospital or of his or her entourage was not carried out in this work.

This study has enabled us to assess the real cost of an embolization procedure, but we would also like to point out a few limitations relating to the sample studied:

- Our small study population of 40 patients.
- Some of the diseases evaluated are represented by a very small number of patients, which does not reflect the true cost of care.

- Follow-up and monitoring of the patient after discharge from NIN are not evaluated in this work, but could be the subject of a follow-up study after embolization.

# CONCLUSION

The pharmacoeconomic study provides a unique tool for evaluating health outcomes in monetary terms and informing healthcare decisions. However, the monetary valuation of health outcomes poses an ethical problem since, ultimately, this method amounts to putting a monetary value on life.

Our study is a pharmacoeconomic evaluation of interventional neuroradiology procedures for cerebro-medullary vascular pathologies.

The objectives of this study were to assess the total cost of an endovascular procedure, to identify its determinants and to compare it with the lump sums allocated by the CNAM.

An embolization procedure costs the National Institute of Neurology between 7,079 DT and 36,325 DT, with a median of 14,046 DT.

The cost of pharmaceuticals accounted for the bulk of overall costs (95.8%), and was dominated by the cost of medical devices used during the procedure (92%), particularly coils, embolic agents and microcatheters.

The majority of neurovascular pathologies treated were aneurysms (n=29). Aneurysm characteristics (aneurysm sac and neck size) and the number of coils used were considered factors influencing variation in the total cost of the procedure, with a significant p-value $< 0.05$.

Although endovascular treatment is generally more costly in terms of medical devices, this increase is more than offset by the savings made in terms of complications, hospitalization time and costs. The advantages of endovascular treatment are numerous, not least for the patient, who benefits from faster recovery, shorter hospital stay, less pain and fewer complications in the post-operative period. Return to professional or personal activities is also quicker than after neurosurgical intervention.

The management of neurovascular pathologies has changed considerably over the last fifteen years. Previously treated exclusively by surgery, they are now increasingly managed by interventional neuroradiology. Developments in medical device technology and the reduced risk of these treatments could make the management of these neuroradiological pathologies even more effective.

## REFERENCES

1. **Rousseau H, Vernhet-Kovacsik H, Mouroz PR, Otal P, Meyrignac O, Mokrane FZ.** Future of interventional radiology. *Presse Med. 2019;48:648-54.*

2. **Beckett JS, Duckwiler GR, Tateshima S, Szeder V, Jahan R, Gonzalez N, et al.**Coil embolization through the Marathon microcatheter: Advantages and pitfalls. *IntervNeuroradiol. 2017;23:28-33.*

3. **Molyneux AJ, Kerr RS, Yu LM, Clarke M, Sneade M, Yarnold JA, et al.** International subarachnoid aneurysm trial (ISAT) of neurosurgical clipping versus endovascular coiling in 2143 patients with ruptured intracranial aneurysms: a randomised comparison of effects on survival, dependency, seizures, rebleeding, subgroups, and aneurysm occlusion. *Lancet 2005;366:809-17.*

4. **Wiebers DO, Whisnant JP, Huston J 3<sup>rd</sup> , Meissner I, Brown RD Jr, Piepgras DG, et al.** Unruptured intracranial aneurysms: natural history, clinical outcome, and risks of surgical and endovascular treatment. *Lancet. 2003;362:103-10.*

5. **Brown RD, Flemming KD, Meyer FB, Cloft HJ, Pollock BE, Link MJ.** Natural history, evaluation, and management of intracranial vascular malformations. *Mayo Clin Proc. 2005;80:26981-.*

6. **Solomon RA, Connolly ES.** Arteriovenous malformations of the brain. *N Engl J Med. 2017;376:185966-.*

7. **Rousseau H, Vernhet-Kovacsik H, Mouroz PR, Otal P, Meyrignac O, Mokrane FZ.** Future of interventional radiology. *Presse Med. 2019;48:648-54.*

8. **Rodesch G, Picard L, Berenstein A, Biondi A, Bracard S, Choi IS, et al.**Interventionalneuroradiology: a neuroscience sub-specialty?.*IntervNeuroradiol. 2013;19:263-70.*

9.  **Hu J, Albadawi H, Chong BW, Deipolyi AR, Sheth RA, Khademhosseini A, et al.**Advances in biomaterials and technologies for vascular embolization. *Adv Mater. 2019;31:e1901071.*

10. **Thuillier L.** Endovascular treatment of middle cerebral artery aneurysms: retrospective study of 202 aneurysms [Thesis]. *Nancy: Université de Lorraine, Faculté de Médecine; 2002.*

11. **Arnold MJ, Keung JJ, McCarragher B.** Interventional radiology: indications and best practices. *IntervRadiol. 2019;99:10.*

12. **Grugeaux M, Bernard L, Charpille D, Mazen J, Gabrillargues D, Boïko-Alaux V, et al.** Interventional neuroradiology: medical devices used according to pathologies. *[Online]. 2009 [Accessed 03/19/2021]. Available: https://www.euro-pharmat.com/communications-affichees/download/3212/3102/170*

13. **Zhou S, Dion PA, Rouleau GA.** Genetics of intracranial aneurysms. *Stroke. 2018;49:780-7.*

14. **Memphis Vascular Center.** Brain Aneurysms. *[Online]. 2021 [Accessed 03/19/2021]. Available: https://memphisvascular.com/patient-education/ brain-aneurysms/*

15. **Sforza DM, Putman CM, Cebral JR.**Hemodynamics of cerebral aneurysms. *Annu Rev Fluid Mech. 2009;41:91-107.*

16. **Schievink WI.** Intracranial Aneurysms. *N Engl J Med. 1997;336:2840-.*

17. **Signorelli F, Sela S, Gesualdo L, Chevrel S, Tollet F, Pailler-Mattei C, et al.**Hemodynamic stress, inflammation, and intracranial aneurysm development and rupture: a systematic review. *World Neurosurg. 2018;115:234-44.*

18. **Yanaka K, Nagase S, Asakawa H, Matsumaru Y, Koyama A, Nose T.** Management of unruptured cerebral aneurysms in patients with polycystic kidney disease. *Surg Neurol. 2004;62:538-45.*

19. **Bowles E.** Cerebral aneurysm and aneurysmal subarachnoid haemorrhage. *Nurs Stand. 2014;28:529-.*

20. **Brisman JL, Song JK, Newell DW.** Cerebral aneurysms. *N Engl J Med. 2006;355:928-39.*

21. **Anxionnat R, Tonnelet R, Derelle AL, Liao L, Barbier C, Bracard S.** Endovascular treatment of ruptured intracranial aneurysms. *J RadiolDiagnInterv. 2015;96:22331-.*

22. **Houdart E.** Coils in interventional neuroradiology. *LettNeurol. 2003;7(9):1-2.*

23. **SCTIMST.** DM Neurology program. *[Online]. 2020 [Accessed 03/19/2021]. Available: https://www.sctimst.ac.in/academic%20and%20research/Academic/ Board%20of%20Studies/resources/DM_Neurology_BOS.pdf*

24. **Picard L, Bracard S, Anxionnatl R, Pradal E, Perez A, Burdin D, et al.** Endovascular treatment of intracranial aneurysms. *Ann Fr AnesthReanim 1996;15:348-53.*

25. **Taylor G, Blanc R, Devys JM.** Anesthesia in interventional neuroradiology: treatment of intracranial aneurysms. *Prat AnesthReanim. 2009;13:32631-.*

26. **Pierot L, Cognard C, Spelle L, Moret J.** Safety and efficacy of balloon remodeling technique during endovascular treatment of intracranial aneurysms: critical review of the literature. *AJNR Am J Neuroradiol. 2012;33:-125.*

27. **Moret J, Cognard C, Weill A, Castaings L, Rey A. The "Remodelling** Technique" in the treatment of wide neck intracranial aneurysms: angiographic results and clinical follow-up in 56 cases. *IntervNeuroradiol. 1997;3:-2135.*

28. **Chung J, Lim YC, Suh SH, Shim YS, Kim YB, Joo JY, et al.** Stent-assisted coil embolization of ruptured wide-necked aneurysms in the acute period: incidence of and risk factors for periprocedural complications. *J Neurosurg. 2014;121:411-.*

29. **Anxionnat R, Tonnelet R, Derelle AL, Liao L, Barbier C, Bracard S.** Endovascular treatment of ruptured intracranial aneurysms. *J RadiolDiagnInterv. 2015;96:22331-.*

30. **Boullery C.** Cerebral aneurysm treatments. *[Online]. 2019 [Accessed 03/19/2021]. Available: http://anevrisme.info/traitements-anevrisme.htm*

31. **Friedlander RM.** Clinical practice. Arteriovenous malformations of the brain. *N Engl J Med. 2007;356:2704-12.*

32. **Barreau X, Marnat G, Gariel F, Dousset V.** Intracranialarteriovenous malformations. *DiagnInterv Imaging. 2014;95:117586-.*

33. **Mayo Clinic.**Arteriovenous malformation.*[Online]. 2021 [Accessed 03/19/2021]. Available: https://www.mayoclinic.org/diseases-conditions/arteriovenous-malformation/symptoms-causes/syc-20350544*

34. **Guimaraes M, Wooster M. Onyx (ethylene-vinyl alcohol copolymer) in** peripheral applications. *SeminIntervRadiol. 2011;28:-3506.*

35. **Mounayer C, Hammami N, Piotin M, Spelle L, Benndorf G, Kessler I, et al.** Nidal embolization of brain arteriovenous malformations using Onyx in 94 patients. *AJNR Am J Neuroradiol. 2007;28:51823-.*

36. **Hill H, Beecham Chick JF, Hage A, Srinivasa RN.** N-butyl cyanoacrylate embolotherapy: techniques, complications, and management. *DiagnIntervRadiol. 2018;24:98-103.*

37. **Matsumoto T, Imagama S, Miyachi S, Izumi T, Matsui H, Muramoto A, et al.**Treatment of perimedullary arteriovenous fistula of the spinal cord by superselectiveneuroendovascular therapy: A case report and literature review. *J OrthopSci. 2016;21:86-90.*

38. **Khouadja S, Younes S, Kacem HH, Arbi F, Sfar MH.** Perimedullary arteriovenous fistula: about a case. *RevNeurol (Paris). 2016;172:A1301-.*

39. **Flores BC, Klinger DR, White JA, Batjer HH.** Spinal vascular malformations: treatment strategies and outcome. *Neurosurg Rev. 2017;40:1528-.*

40. **Sacco RL, Kasner SE, Broderick JP, Caplan LR, Connors JJ, Culebras A, et al.** An updated definition of stroke for the 21st century: a statement for healthcare professionals from the American Heart Association/American Stroke Association. *Stroke. 2013;44:2064-89.*

41. **Liaw N, Liebeskind D.** Emerging therapies in acute ischemic stroke. *F1000Res. 2020;9:546.*

42. **Gory B, Laprgue B.** Place of mechanical thrombectomy in ischemic stroke in the postoperative period. *Prat AnesthReanim. 2018;22:88-92.*

43. **Haute Autorité de Santé.** Endovascular thrombectomy of intracranial arteries. *Paris: HAS; 2016.*

44. **Bonafe A, Costalat V, Machi P, Riquelme C, Eker O, Menjot De Champfleur S, et al**. Place of mechanical thrombectomy in the treatment of acute stroke. *Prat Neurol FMC. 2013;4:936-.*

45. **Attye A, Boubagra K, Grand S, Heck O, Kastler A, Krainik A, et al.**Mechanical thrombectomy in the management of acute ischemic stroke.*[Online]. 2018 [Accessed 03/19/2021]. Available: https://www.chu-grenoble.fr/content/thrombectomie-mecanique-dans-la-prise-en-charge-des-avc-ischemiques-aigus*

46. **Turk AS, Spiotta A, Frei D, Mocco J, Baxter B, Fiorella D, et al.** Initial clinical experience with the ADAPT technique: A direct aspiration first pass technique for stroke thrombectomy. *J Neurointerv Surg. 2018;10(Suppl 1):20-5.*

47. **Crochard-Lacour A, LeLorier J.** Introduction to pharmacoeconomics. *Montreal QC: Presses de l'Université de Montréal; 2016.*

48. **Losser M, Payen D.** Meningeal hemorrhage: management. *Reanimation. 2007;16:46371-.*

49. **Garattini L, Tediosi F, Ghislandi S, Orzella L, Rossi C.** How do Italian pharmacoeconomists evaluate indirect costs? *Value health. 2000;3:2706-.*

50. **Woronoff-Lemsi MC, Limat S, Husson MC.** Pharmaco-economic approach and illustrations in hospital settings. *J Pharm Clin. 2000;19:53-8.*

51. **Bekelis K, Missios S, Labropoulos N.** Cerebral aneurysm coiling: a predictive model of hospitalization cost. *J NeuroInterventional Surg. 2015;7:5438-.*

52. **Zubair Tahir M, Enam SA, Pervez Ali R, Bhatti A, Ul Haq T.** Cost-effectiveness of clipping vs coiling of intracranial aneurysms after subarachnoid hemorrhage in a developing country: a prospective study. *Surg Neurol. 2009;72:35560-.*

53. **Cheikh A, El Abbadi N, Ismaïli H, Ababou A, Cherrah Y, El Quessar A.** The cost of management of intracranial aneurysms by embolization in Morocco: About 48 cases. *Int J Pharm Sci. 2014;6:8226-.*

54. **Labalette C, Houdart E, David S, Rymer R, Duteil C, Tacnet JF, et al.** Embolization of cerebral aneurysms: funding developments and outlook. *J Radiol. 2010;91(9 Pt 1):895-900.*

55. **Cheikh A, Rachid R, Jehanne A, Adil A, Ali B, Cherrah Y, et al.** Cost of treatment of cerebral aneurysm embolization: study of associated factors. *NeurolTher. 2016;5:145-54.*

56. **Qureshi AI, Luft AR, Sharma M, Guterman LR, Hopkins LN.** Prevention and treatment of thromboembolic and ischemic complications associated with endovascular procedures. Part II: Clinical aspects and recommendations. *Neurosurgery. 2000;46:136076-.*

57. **Mejdoubi M, Gigaud M, Trémoulet M, Albucher JF, Cognard C.** Initial primary endovascular treatment in the management of ruptured intracranial aneurysms: a prospective consecutive series. *Neuroradiology. 2006;48:-899905.*

58. **Ozpar R, Nas OF, Hacikurt K, Taskapilioglu MO, Kocaeli H, Hakyemez B.** Endovascular treatment of intracranial arteriovenous malformations using detachable-tip microcatheters and Onyx 18$^®$ . *DiagnInterv Imaging. 2019;100:353-61.*

59. **Sluzewski M, Bosch JA, van Rooij WJ, Nijssen PC, Wijnalda D.** Rupture of intracranial aneurysms during treatment with Guglielmi detachable coils: incidence, outcome, and risk factors. *J Neurosurg. 2001;94:23840-.*

60. **Houdart E.** Complications of embolization in interventional neuroradiology. *LettNeurol 2005;9:153-8.*

61. **Elewa MK.** Endovascular coiling for cerebral aneurysm: single-center experience in Egypt. *Egypt J NeurolPsychiatrNeurosurg. 2018;54:33.*

62. **Twitchell S, Abou-Al-Shaar H, Reese J, Karsy M, Eli IM, Guan J, et al.** Analysis of cerebrovascular aneurysm treatment cost: retrospective cohort comparison of clipping, coiling, and flow diversion. *Neurosurg Focus. 2018;44:E3.*

63. **Spetzler RF, Albuquerque FC, Partovi S.** The barrow ruptured aneurysm trial: 3-year results. *J Neurosurg. 2013;119:12.*

64. **Ballet AC, Guérin J, Berge J, Taboulet F, Martin S, Philip V, et al.** Neurosurgical and endovascular treatment of intracranial aneurysms. An economic approach to two therapeutic alternatives at Bordeaux University Hospital. *Neurosurgery. 2002;48:419-25.*

65. **Lad SP, Babu R, Rhee MS, Franklin RL, Ugiliweneza B, Hodes J, et al.** Long-term economic impact of coiling vs clipping for unruptured intracranial aneurysms. *Neurosurgery. 2013;72:100013-.*

66. **Spetzler RF, McDougall CG, Zabramski JM, Albuquerque FC, Hills NK, Russin JJ, et al.** The barrowrupturedaneurysm trial: 6-year results. *J Neurosurg. 2015;123:609-17.*

67. **Pierot L, Cognard C, Anxionnat R, Ricolfi F; CLARITY Investigators.** Endovascular treatment of ruptured intracranial aneurysms: factors affecting midterm quality anatomic results: analysis in a prospective, multicenter series of patients (CLARITY). *AJNR Am J Neuroradiol. 2012;33:1475-80.*

68. **Rutledge C, Nelson J, Lu A, Nisson P, Jonzzon S, Winkler EA, et al.** Cost determinants in management of brain arteriovenous malformations. *ActaNeurochir (Wien). 2020;162:16973-.*

69. **Miller CE, Quayyum Z, McNamee P, Al-Shahi Salman R.** Economic burden of intracranial vascular malformations in adults: prospective population-based study. *Stroke. 2009;40:19739-.*

70. **Balami JS, Coughlan D, White PM, McMeekin P, Flynn D, Roffe C, et al.** The cost of providing mechanical thrombectomy in the UK NHS: a micro-costing study. *Clin Med. 2020;20(3):e405-.*

71. **Wahlgren N, Moreira T, Michel P, Steiner T, Jansen O, Cognard C, et al.** Mechanical thrombectomy in acute ischemic stroke: Consensus statement by ESO-Karolinska Stroke Update 2014/2015, supported by ESO, ESMINT, ESNR and EAN. *Int J Stroke. 2016;11:13447-.*

# APPENDIX

# Data collection form

**Patient information:***File no.*: ..................
- Full name:
...............................................................................................................................

- Gender: Male ☐ Female ☐

- Age
:...............................................................................................................................
...................

- Profession:
...............................................................................................................................
.....

- Comorbidities:
...............................................................................................................................

- Type of social security coverage: CNAM ☐ Indigent ☐ Other: .......................................

- Place of residence:
...............................................................................................................................

- Means of transport and cost:
.............................................................................................................

- Travel accommodation and costs:
....................................................................................


**Diagnosis :**
- Aneurysm ☐

☐ **Qualifying the** ☐ Size:
  **aneurysm**
.............................................................. Neck size:............................................

Ruptured☐Not ruptured

- MAV ☐

-FAV ☐

- Ischemic stroke ☐


**Interventional neuroradiology management :**
- Date of intervention: ....................................................

**- Medications used during the procedure :**

| DCI | Quantity | | DCI | Quantity |
|---|---|---|---|---|
| | | | | |
| | | | | |
| | | | | |
| | | | | |
| | | | | |
| | | | | |
| | | | | |
| | | | | |

**- Medical devices used during the procedure :**

| Designation | Quantity | | Designation | Quantity |
|---|---|---|---|---|
| | | | | |
| | | | | |
| | | | | |
| | | | | |
| | | | | |
| | | | | |
| | | | | |
| | | | | |
| | | | | |
| | | | | |

-Depreciation of intervention room: ................................

## Hospitalization :

- Total hospital stay: ................

- Hospitalization department: Intensive care ☐Other departments ☐

- Absenteeism: ........................... and impact on patient pay: .......................

- Evolution : Alive ☐Deceased ☐

**- Medications used during hospitalization :**

| DCI | Quantity/day | |
|---|---|---|

|  | J0 | J1 | J2 | J3 | J4 | J5 | J6 | J7 | J8 | J9 | J10 | J11 | J12 | J13 | **Total quantity** |
|---|---|---|---|---|---|---|---|---|---|---|---|---|---|---|---|
|  |  |  |  |  |  |  |  |  |  |  |  |  |  |  |  |
|  |  |  |  |  |  |  |  |  |  |  |  |  |  |  |  |
|  |  |  |  |  |  |  |  |  |  |  |  |  |  |  |  |
|  |  |  |  |  |  |  |  |  |  |  |  |  |  |  |  |
|  |  |  |  |  |  |  |  |  |  |  |  |  |  |  |  |
|  |  |  |  |  |  |  |  |  |  |  |  |  |  |  |  |
|  |  |  |  |  |  |  |  |  |  |  |  |  |  |  |  |
|  |  |  |  |  |  |  |  |  |  |  |  |  |  |  |  |
|  |  |  |  |  |  |  |  |  |  |  |  |  |  |  |  |

**- Medical devices used during hospitalization :**

| **Designation** | **Quantity/day** | | | | | | | | | | | | | | **Total quantity** |
|---|---|---|---|---|---|---|---|---|---|---|---|---|---|---|---|
|  | J0 | J1 | J2 | J3 | J4 | J5 | J6 | J7 | J8 | J9 | J10 | J11 | J12 | J13 |  |
|  |  |  |  |  |  |  |  |  |  |  |  |  |  |  |  |
|  |  |  |  |  |  |  |  |  |  |  |  |  |  |  |  |
|  |  |  |  |  |  |  |  |  |  |  |  |  |  |  |  |
|  |  |  |  |  |  |  |  |  |  |  |  |  |  |  |  |
|  |  |  |  |  |  |  |  |  |  |  |  |  |  |  |  |
|  |  |  |  |  |  |  |  |  |  |  |  |  |  |  |  |

## Complications: Yes ☐ No ☐

- Complication type: ................................................................................................................

- Additional hospital stay: ...........................................

**- Medications used after the complication :**

| **DCI** | **Quantity/day** |  |
|---|---|---|

| | J0 | J1 | J2 | J3 | J4 | J5 | J6 | J7 | J8 | J9 | J10 | J11 | J12 | J13 | Total quantity |
|---|---|---|---|---|---|---|---|---|---|---|---|---|---|---|---|
| | | | | | | | | | | | | | | | |
| | | | | | | | | | | | | | | | |
| | | | | | | | | | | | | | | | |
| | | | | | | | | | | | | | | | |
| | | | | | | | | | | | | | | | |
| | | | | | | | | | | | | | | | |
| | | | | | | | | | | | | | | | |
| | | | | | | | | | | | | | | | |
| | | | | | | | | | | | | | | | |

**- Medical devices used after the complication :**

| Designation | Quantity/day | | | | | | | | | | | | | | Total quantity |
|---|---|---|---|---|---|---|---|---|---|---|---|---|---|---|---|
| | J0 | J1 | J2 | J3 | J4 | J5 | J6 | J7 | J8 | J9 | J10 | J11 | J12 | J13 | |
| | | | | | | | | | | | | | | | |
| | | | | | | | | | | | | | | | |
| | | | | | | | | | | | | | | | |
| | | | | | | | | | | | | | | | |
| | | | | | | | | | | | | | | | |
| | | | | | | | | | | | | | | | |
| | | | | | | | | | | | | | | | |

**Additional tests :**

(From date of intervention J0: ...............................................)

- X-rays: / patient

| Different types of Rx | Length of hospital stay | | | | | | | | | | | | | | Total quantity |
|---|---|---|---|---|---|---|---|---|---|---|---|---|---|---|---|
| | J0 | J1 | J2 | J3 | J4 | J5 | J6 | J7 | J8 | J9 | J10 | J11 | J12 | J13 | |
| | | | | | | | | | | | | | | | |
| | | | | | | | | | | | | | | | |
| | | | | | | | | | | | | | | | |
| | | | | | | | | | | | | | | | |
| | | | | | | | | | | | | | | | |
| | | | | | | | | | | | | | | | |
| | | | | | | | | | | | | | | | |
| | | | | | | | | | | | | | | | |
| | | | | | | | | | | | | | | | |
| | | | | | | | | | | | | | | | |
| | | | | | | | | | | | | | | | |
| | | | | | | | | | | | | | | | |

-Biology: / patient

| Different types of balance sheet | Length of hospital stay | | | | | | | | | | | | | | Total quantity |
|---|---|---|---|---|---|---|---|---|---|---|---|---|---|---|---|
| | J0 | J1 | J2 | J3 | J4 | J5 | J6 | J7 | J8 | J9 | J10 | J11 | J12 | J13 | |
| | | | | | | | | | | | | | | | |
| | | | | | | | | | | | | | | | |
| | | | | | | | | | | | | | | | |
| | | | | | | | | | | | | | | | |
| | | | | | | | | | | | | | | | |
| | | | | | | | | | | | | | | | |

83

# ANTI-PLAGIARISM CHARTER

At the request of the Commission des Thèses de Doctorat en Pharmacie and the Conseil Scientifique, the Faculté de Pharmacie de Monastir has embarked on a policy to combat plagiarism. This policy includes raising awareness of the seriousness of this criminal practice among all staff and students.

Students enrolled at the Faculty of Pharmacy of Monastir undertake to respect the rules of intellectual honesty set out in the anti-plagiarism charter.

## 1. General definitions

Plagiarism: "The act of someone who, in the artistic or literary field what he has taken from the work of another", Le Larousse.

Plagiarism occurs when you directly copy the work of others (including on the Internet) without indicating this borrowing in the form of a duly referenced quotation.

Plagiarism may concern the entire work submitted, or one or more parts of it. No matter how much or how little of the work is taken from others, sanctions will be applied as decided by of the Faculty of Pharmacy. Plagiarism must therefore be understood as a legal infringement of the rules governing respect for copyright in accordance with Decree no. 2008-2422 of June 23, 2008 (JORT).

## 2. Responsibilities

Having received the present charter, students are considered to be entirely responsible for the work they produce, its scientific content and the originality of their thinking.

## 3. Commitments

Students undertake to cite the works they use or partially reproduce, in compliance with the rules set out in the thesis guide.

The methodology for writing a Doctor of Pharmacy thesis requires that borrowings be clearly identified and that the author's name and the source of the extract be mentioned.

## 4. Sanctions

Plagiarism is severely punished at the Faculty of Pharmacy in Monastir. Any student caught in the act of plagiarism risks having his or her thesis rejected, not being awarded the Doctor of Pharmacy diploma, and being banned from taking part in any competitive examination organized by the Ministry of Higher Education, Scientific Research and Technology for 5 consecutive years.

I, TrakiMazouni, acknowledge that I have read this charter and agree to abide by its principles.

June 18, 2021                                    Signature

# FINAL VALIDATION

## CADRE RESERVE A LA COMMISSION DE THESE

Ce manuscrit a été examiné par un membre de la commission de thèse qui atteste par la présente que:

☐ Cette copie du manuscrit a reçu un avis favorable pour la soutenance.

☐ Cette copie du manuscrit est conforme à la copie examinée initialement par la Commission et ayant reçu un avis favorable pour la soutenance.

☐ La date prévue pour la soutenance est fixée dans un délai minimum de 10 jours à partir de ce jour.

Date: .......................................Nom           -          Prénom:

.............................................

Signature

## CADRE RESERVE AU PRESIDENT DU JURY
### (à remplir si jugé nécessaire lors de la soutenance)

☐ Cette copie de la thèse comporte toutes les modifications effectuées après la soutenance selon les recommandations des membres du jury.

Date: .......................................Nom           -          Prénom:

.............................................

Signature

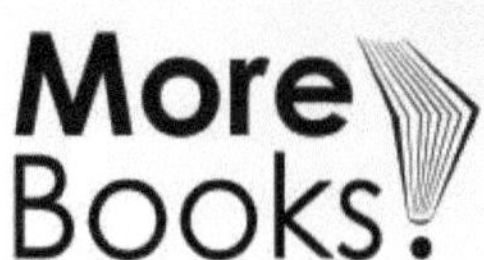
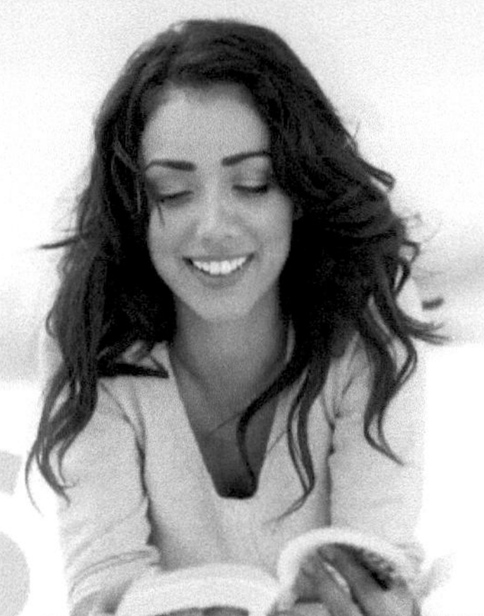

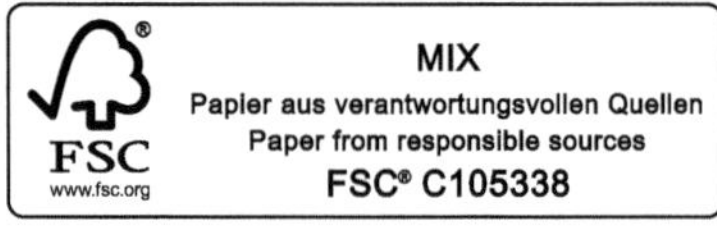

Printed by Books on Demand GmbH, Norderstedt / Germany